Praise for
Never Feel Old Again

"Raymond Francis adds another excellent book to his previous masterpieces. This is a powerful formula for health that should remain in one's library for frequent reference. It is one of the most sensible books on maintaining health and avoiding frailty of old age I have ever seen. We all owe Raymond Francis a note of gratitude for this wonderful book."

Russell L. Blaylock, MD, CCN
Theoretical Neuroscience Research, LLC,
author, *Natural Strategies for Cancer Patients,*
Health and Nutrition Secrets that Can Save Your Life,
and *Excitotoxins: The Taste That Kills,*
www.blaylockwellnesscenter.com

"While reading this book, I was reminded of the Satchel Paige quote, 'How old would you be if you didn't know how old you are?' This book will show you how to BE much younger than your years for the rest of your life."

J. Morris Hicks
consultant; author of *Healthy Eating, Healthy World,*
and international blogger, *www.hpjmh.com*

"Raymond Francis has written an outstanding, groundbreaking book on slowing the aging process. In a thoughtful, comprehensive way, he simplifies complex issues and offers practical advice on how to stay biologically young and vigorous.

"This book is a user-friendly, commonsense, practical guide to living a longer healthier life and should be read by everyone who is concerned about aging."

David Rovno, MD
Distinguished Life Fellow of the American
Psychiatric Association, former Assistant
Clinical Professor, UCSF School of Medicine

"*Never Feel Old Again* cuts through the confusion and provides the keys that unlock the mysteries of the aging process. Raymond Francis in his simple and compelling style shows us now it is possible to take control of our health and reduce our biological age. A must-read for everyone who is aging and wants to maximize their youthfulness!"

Len Saputo, MD
Author of *A Return to Healing*
www.doctorsaputo.com

"Raymond Francis is the real deal. There is some great information in this book that will make a difference for everyone who takes it to heart."

Frank Shallenberger, MD
Editor, *Real Cures Newsletter*
Medical Director, The Nevada Center
for Anti-Aging Medicine

"*Never Feel Old Again* is an eye opener to help people learn about health, make better choices, and to live longer, higher-quality lives. You don't have to feel old!"

Bernd Friedlander, DC
Care Wellness Center
San Mateo, CA

Never Feel Old Again

Aging Is a Mistake— Learn How to Avoid It

Raymond Francis

Health Communications, Inc.
Deerfield Beach, Florida

www.hcibooks.com

Disclaimer: This book and the advice contained herein are not intended to be used as a substitute for the advice and/or medical care of the reader's physician, nor are they intended to discourage or dissuade the reader from the advice of his or her physician. The reader should regularly consult with a physician in matters relating to his or her health, especially with regard to symptoms that may require diagnosis. Any eating, exercise, or lifestyle regimen should not be undertaken without first consulting the reader's physician.

Library of Congress Cataloging-in-Publication Data

Francis, Raymond, 1937-
    Never feel old again / Raymond Francis.
        pages cm
    ISBN-13: 978-0-7573-1732-3 (Paperback)
    ISBN-10: 0-7573-1732-4 (Paperback)
    ISBN-13: 978-0-7573-1733-0 (ePub)
    ISBN 0-7573-1733-2 (ePub)
    1. Longevity.   2. Aging—Prevention.   3. Older people—Health and hygiene.
    4. Self-care, Health.   I. Title.
    RA776.75.F733 2013
    613.2—dc23

                                                                2013016719

Publisher: Health Communications, Inc.
        3201 S.W. 15th Street
        Deerfield Beach, FL 33442–8190

Cover image ©Dreamstime.com
Cover design by Larissa Hise Henoch
Interior design and formatting by Lawna Patterson Oldfield

CONTENTS

ACKNOWLEDGMENTS

THIS BOOK IS THE CULMINATION OF almost thirty years of learning and experience. It is impossible to write such a work without the support of others, and I would like to take this opportunity to acknowledge and thank all those who contributed to the creation and production of this book. In addition to all the great thinkers, researchers, and practitioners who created the knowledge upon which this book is based, numerous other people have helped to make the book a reality as well as more readable, relevant, and useful to the reader. I want to acknowledge and express my appreciation to everyone who contributed in any capacity.

Special thanks go to my talented editor, Norman Hawker, who is always there when you need him, and whose valuable contributions are too many to list. Thanks also for meaningful contributions from Richardine O'Brien, Pamela Strong, Jeanelle Viola, Kelly Florko, Joan Carole, Austin Jett, Richard Higgins, Robin Organ, and Dr. David Rovno.

Lastly, I want to thank my wonderful publisher, Health Communications, Inc. (HCI), for making this book possible and for their many contributions to making the world a better place. Thanks also to my HCI editor, Allison Janse, for her years of friendship, patient guidance, and encouragement.

FOREWORD

You Don't Have to Be Sick If You Take Responsibility for Your Health

A S I WRITE THIS, POPE BENEDICT XVI has resigned from the papal office, becoming the first pope to do so in nearly 700 years. His resignation sent shock waves throughout the world and has been attributed to his worsening health problems.

Pope Benedict is 85 years old. Sadly, his failing health is the norm for so many senior citizens today, as well as for much of our population in general. In fact, it's commonly accepted by the majority of people today that illness and eventual decrepitude is part and parcel of growing older. And with very good reason, for there is no question that the incidence of disease and disabilities increases with each passing decade of life for most people who are alive today throughout the Western world. As a result, in the United States alone, sales of prescription drugs account for over 13 percent of our nation's health care expenditures, with the majority of those sales being made to men and women who are 50 and older. Consider these shocking statistics:

62 percent of all Americans incur annual expenses for prescription
drugs.

And among people age 65 or older, that rate jumps up to a
whopping 90 percent!

And that's just the tip of the iceberg. In his book, *Generation Rx:
How Prescription Drugs Are Altering American Lives, Minds,
and Bodies*, author Greg Critser cites the following facts:

The average number of prescriptions drugs used per person, per
year, in 1993 was seven.

The average number of prescriptions drugs used per person, per
year, in 2000 was eleven.

The average number of prescriptions drugs used per person, per
year, in 2004 was twelve.

Mr. Critser published his book in 2005. Since that time, the
figures above have likely risen even further. Clearly there is something seriously wrong with this picture. Especially given the fact
that, despite the enormous amount of money spent on health care
costs in the U.S. each year, as a nation we continue to get sicker
and sicker and now rank at the bottom of the health index of
industrialized nations.

As I mentioned, most people today blindly shrug off these facts
under the mistaken belief that "That's simply the way life goes; as
we get older we get sicker and our health costs rise as well."

I'm here to tell that they are wrong. Not only do you NOT have
to get sicker as you age, *you can become even healthier than you
were when you were younger.*

I'm living proof of this fact.

I am a year older than Pope Benedict. As he was announcing his retirement, I was enjoying an active vacation skiing in Europe. In another week, I will again be hitting the ski slopes, this time in Aspen, Colorado. As I have aged, my health markers have actually improved. I continue to enjoy a healthy sex life; I frequently travel throughout the world, presenting lectures on health and longevity; and while most of my peers (the ones who are still alive, that is), have long since retired, I continue to explore new business ventures while keeping abreast of the latest breakthroughs and research across the wide field of medicine, both conventional and integrative and alternative.

What is my secret?

I don't have one. Instead, I can tell you that the reason I remain vitally healthy is because, more than forty-five years ago, I realized how important it was for me to take responsibility for my health and well-being. Since that time, by following the precepts and using the therapies that I have covered so extensively in my many books, I have been blessed with greater health and energy.

In the course of my health journey, I have also learned that, in the United States as well as in many other nations, we are poisoning ourselves to death. Our air, soil, and water supplies continue to be polluted with harmful toxins. Our food supplies continue to show a decline in their nutritive value due to the ongoing loss of minerals in our croplands, the widespread use of harmful pesticides, preservatives, and other chemicals to grow, harvest, and transport food, and the unnatural ways that we now produce fish, poultry meat, and dairy products. Similarly, our water supplies also face an ongoing onslaught of unhealthy chemicals and other toxins. And, as if that is not enough, now we are faced with the growing use of genetically modified "Frankenfood crops" and even genetically modified fish and other foods, despite the fact that no long-term safety studies have ever been conducted for such abominations, and animal studies already show that such "foods" greatly increase the risk of cancer and other diseases.

You might think that our government needs to step in and right these very serious wrongs. If so, you are correct. But don't count on it anytime soon. Why? Because our government is wholly owned and operated today by powerful special influences, including the Big Pharma, Big Agriculture, Big Medicine, Big Chemical, and the nuclear power cartels, all of which care for their ever increasing profit margins at the expense of our health and the health of our environment.

Meanwhile, it is up to you and me and everyone else to do all that we can to take control of our own health. For many people, this means relying on their doctors. I disagree. Why? Because most doctors today, despite their many years of education and training, don't have a clue about what it means to be healthy, let alone what is required to achieve and maintain optimal health. Regardless of how educated they may be, when it comes to achieving health, the average doctor today is virtually worthless. Did you know, for example, that in their eight years of medical school, doctors only receive a total of twenty-five hours of nutritional education? That's less than one week. You can easily exceed what they know about nutrition simply by reading a few books, starting with the one you now hold in your hands.

Here's another example of how doctors fail to put two and two together. It has long been proven that cancer cells thrive on sugar as their primary food source. That's why PET scans are able to detect cancerous tumors. As they scan the body, any areas that show tumors light up on the scan because of their higher concentrations of sugar. But do oncologists and other doctors educate their patients about the dangers of sugar? Very rarely, if ever. Instead, many oncologist offices today offer sugar-laden lollipops to child patients, and cookies to their other patients. In short, they don't think. If they did, they would be telling all of their patients that not only do cancer cells survive on sugar, but when cancer patients consume sugar it is the equivalent of putting gasoline on a fire.

Please don't mistake what I am saying here, however. I am certainly not against doctors or the obvious benefits that conventional medicine has to offer. But you must realize that these benefits primarily extend to emergency room and trauma care. For treating acute health issues, conventional medicine is unparalleled and nothing can compete with it when it comes to the surgical advances it has made and continues to make. But don't confuse treating acute health conditions with chronic degenerative disease, which accounts for approximately 85 percent of all health conditions in the United States. For such chronic conditions, conventional doctors are little more than legalized drug pushers, doling out drugs solely to manage symptoms, NOT to address the underlying causes.

In addition, most doctors today pay little, if any, attention to preventing disease before it strikes. Yet the importance of doing so cannot be overemphasized. One of the reasons that I remain vitally healthy is because I regularly have myself screened for signs of disease before it can manifest. I do this via a range of medical tests ranging from blood and hormone tests to diagnostic methods based on quantum physics, such as electrodermal screening. Plus I also use anti-aging measures, including a stem cell product derived from sheep placentas that has made a dramatic difference in my health.

But even if doctors were more aware about the most important factors related to health, we still can't count on them to be there for us because today they are forced to spend less than five minutes with their patients in consultation, and growing numbers of doctors are so disenchanted with how unrewarding their profession has become for them that they are leaving it in droves. As a result, studies both within and outside the medical community reveal that within the next five years or so we will be facing a severe shortage of doctors, as well as nurses and other health care professionals.

Simply put, if you desire to become healthier and then to maintain your health gains, there is only one person that you can truly count on—yourself! Like me, you too must take responsibility for your health. The first step, just as it was for me, is to become better educated about health. To that end, I highly recommend this book. It is nothing less than a step-by-step manual that will show you how your body works and what you need to do to get and stay healthy. Like me, its author, Raymond Francis, is a "senior citizen." Also like me, you would never know it. That's because he too, long ago, took responsibility for his health and did everything he needed to do to educate himself about improving and maintaining it. And now he is sharing the fruits of his many years of research with you.

So read on and put what Raymond shares to good use. If you do, you will never again fear a decline in your health and well-being. Instead, the rest of your life will truly become your Golden Years.

God bless,

Burton Goldberg, 2013

Burton Goldberg, often called the voice of alternative medicine, is a leading spokesperson for the rapidly growing field of alternative medicine. He is the author of eighteen books on alternative medicine, including the iconic: Alternative Medicine: The Definitive Guide.

PREFACE

Accelerated Aging Is a Mistake

MY FATHER DIED OF "complications" at age 68.

He was too young to die, but he had already been suffering from diabetes, heart disease, cancer, and high blood pressure for more than a decade. He was filling twelve prescriptions every month. His poor health affected every aspect of his life, depriving him of the basic enjoyments so many of us take for granted. Walking, getting around, and even breathing became increasingly difficult, and dementia was beginning to set in.

Being a wealthy celebrity, I was able to get my dad the best doctors and a spare-no-expense level of medical care—the very best that modern Western medicine could provide. It was not enough.

In fact, I have come to believe that my father's health declined more rapidly *because of* the medical care he received, not *despite* it. Now that I understand how toxic prescription medications are, I no longer wonder why he did so poorly and died so young.

Because of my father's experience, I became resolved to learn as much as I could and take whatever actions would be necessary to prevent suffering a similar fate myself.

In fairness to the medical establishment, they are not the reason my dad had so many illnesses in the first place. However, once these chronic, degenerative diseases took up residence in his body, conventional medicine did nothing that helped and many things that harmed him.

By a stroke of good fortune, I happened to hear Raymond Francis being interviewed on National Public Radio, at a time when my motivation to learn about health was strong. His message was simple: if the cells in your body are healthy, then *you* are healthy, and if the cells are not healthy, then *you* are not healthy. As a scientist, he was taking a common sense look at the true cause of disease and identifying pathways to health that made a lot of sense to me. I decided I had to contact this man, and I am grateful every day that I did.

After reading Raymond's books and being mentored by him, I am in the best health of my life. I simply don't get sick any more— no colds, no flu, or anything else. The allergies I used to suffer all my life are now distant memories. And like Raymond, who is now in his upper seventies, I'm making my organs and blood vessels younger each year. If you read this book and follow Raymond's advice, you will learn how to make your *biological* age younger than your *chronological* age.

The media, the pharmaceutical and health insurance companies, government health agencies, and medical associations would all like us to believe that the "wonders of modern medicine" are helping us to live longer, healthier lives. A realistic appraisal of the facts, however, paints a very different picture. Americans are suffering from an explosion of chronic diseases like diabetes, obesity, cardiovascular disease, cancer, and Alzheimer's disease. The regrettable truth is this: our children may be the first generation that is not expected to live as long as their parents!

As Raymond points out clearly and succinctly, our population is seriously malnourished—not in *calories*, certainly, but in *nutrients*—and our bodies are filled with toxins. Inevitably, the result is an epidemic of poor health. Unfortunately, our response has been a proliferation of medications and medical interventions that are making us sicker and accelerating the aging process. This inappropriate response is the real reason for the healthcare crisis that is pushing our country to the brink of insolvency.

Despite all their claims to the contrary, modern conventional medicine has not cured, and *cannot* cure any disease. Chasing after symptoms does not ferret out the cause, and addressing the cause is the only way to prevent and cure disease.

While the medical establishment is confused by the explosion of chronic disease, rampant childhood diabetes, and illnesses unheard of in our nation's history, Raymond Francis, thankfully, is not one of the confused. Ever since he cured himself of a terminal illness when he was 48 years old, using the principles explained in this book, Raymond has dedicated his life to bringing his "health is a choice" message to as many people as possible. Many thousands have put themselves on the path of wellness after reading

Raymond's other brilliant and easy to follow masterpieces, *Never Be Sick Again*, *Never Be Fat Again*, and *Never Fear Cancer Again*.

Since following Raymond's simple model of health, I have not only vastly improved my own health, but using this knowledge, I have been able to help both friends and family to reverse their cancer, obesity, diabetes, allergies, and arthritis. This book is a continuation of Raymond's outpouring of generosity and love, and his wish for all of us to get well, stay well, and live long disease-free lives. I feel blessed that I opened the door to what Raymond had to say.

This book could be that doorway for you and your loved ones.

To your health,
Rob Schneider
Actor, Comedian, Screenwriter, and Director

INTRODUCTION

Y OU MIGHT BE ASKING YOURSELF, WHAT can this book do for me? Will it provide new and useful information? Can it help me make a change for the better? Will I age any slower? The answer is this book can teach you a unique, science-based model of health, disease, and aging *that will provide you with the keys to controlling the aging process.*

I will explain why we age, and the difference between healthy, normal aging and the disease-filled, accelerated aging most people experience today. I will show you how health and disease really work, and how you can enter your later years confident and in control with the power to enjoy abundant health and vitality until the very end. In short, this book has the potential to transform and enhance your life in ways you may have never dreamed possible.

Why do we fear old age? For most of us, it is not death itself, but "getting old" that stirs a feeling of dread in us. We imagine a life of declining health, a weak and fragile body, diminished mental capacity, and the ultimate indignity of having to depend on others to function on a daily basis. This is an image of a life not worth living—something we would all like to avoid or at least put off as long as possible.

Why then are most of us doing *everything in our power to hasten its arrival*?

That's right. As a culture, we are accelerating the aging process at an alarming rate, and it is costing us immeasurable losses in quality and enjoyment in the later decades of our lives. We develop chronic illnesses like diabetes, heart disease, and arthritis when we should be in good health. We become disabled when we could be capable and strong. Most of us die prematurely of preventable and curable diseases.

Aging this way is a mistake. It is a mistake made moment by moment and day by day throughout our lives. It is a mistake caused by choices made for us as children and choices we make for ourselves as adults. As a result, we now have thirty-year-olds who exhibit biological markers that are typical of eighty-year-olds. Overweight ten-year-olds are showing biological aging that is typical of forty-five-year-olds.

Talk about accelerated aging! If children are biologically forty-five at age ten, what will they be when they are fifty? American children today are so far from optimal health, they are projected to be the first generation in more than two hundred years that will have shorter lives than those of their parents.

Unfortunately, many of us take better care of our cars than we do of our bodies. We wouldn't think of putting salt in the radiator, soybean oil in the engine, or corn syrup in the gas tank. Nor would we drive with the brakes on, switch into reverse while barreling down the highway, or bang into everything that happens to be in our way. Everybody knows that these reckless actions would cause severe damage to a car. Yet, day after day, year after year, many of us are similarly careless in how we treat our bodies.

We load the grocery cart with processed foods, wash down fast food with supersized sodas, suffer increasing levels of stress without an outlet, reach for something—anything—to feel better, stare for hours at one screen or another, and then hit the sack for too few hours of fitful sleep. Few of us realize that living like this for years may be sentencing us to a life of high medical bills, invasive surgeries, and chronic and degenerative diseases, leading to an untimely death. Unlike a car, we can't trash our body and then just get a new one.

If you choose a typical modern diet and lifestyle and do not intend to make any changes, you are choosing the path of accelerated aging and untimely death. However, if you are willing to take a serious look at the way you eat, the way you move, and the way you live, and then make some adjustments, you can in fact achieve total health and never feel old again.

You Can Be Younger than Your Years

You see, it is entirely possible to be *biologically* younger than your *chronological* age, and that is exactly what this book is about. Being biologically younger than your years is easier to achieve than you might think, because *the human body is a self-repairing system*. It is designed to keep you fully functional and in good health for a long lifetime. All you have to do is supply the body with what it needs to keep up its own maintenance. The dreaded symptoms of aging that many of us have come to see as normal are nothing but a disease of repair deficits. A poorly maintained car ends up in a junkyard, and a poorly maintained body ends up in a nursing home.

This does not have to happen to you!

There are entire societies, such as the Himalayan Hunzas and the Japanese Okinawans, who have been able to enjoy excellent health and vitality into an advanced old age. There are also many individuals who achieve this, regardless of the culture around them.

One outstanding example is Jack LaLanne, an icon of modern physical fitness. LaLanne set out to prove that age was no obstacle to great physical performance. He ate a healthy diet and exercised every day of his life, until he died in 2011 at age ninety-six. He drew worldwide attention for swimming from Alcatraz Island to Fisherman's Wharf in San Francisco at age sixty while handcuffed, shackled, and pulling a thousand-pound boat. At age seventy, he towed seventy boats carrying seventy people through Long Beach Harbor while handcuffed and shackled once again.

I myself am in my mid-seventies, but I am in excellent shape both physically and mentally. My arteries, and the medical odds of my having a heart attack or stroke, match those of a man in his mid-twenties. I never get sick. I have had only two colds in the last twenty-seven years. I have no arthritis, no hip or knee replacements, and no artificial implements anywhere in my body. I have no cataracts or macular degeneration in my eyes. I take no drugs. I am mentally sharp and full of energy. Do you remember being a kid and having so much energy you didn't know what to do with it all? That's how I feel at seventy-six.

How This Book Can Help You

In this book, I will show you how to take control of your health and reduce your biological age. Virtually all aging our society experiences today is premature. Yet premature aging is not natural or inevitable; it is a disease of deferred maintenance. In fact, I will explain that, regardless of symptoms, there really is only one disease, and that this one disease only has two causes. I will teach you how to control these two causes of aging and disease through the Six Pathways to health or disease.

Approaching aging as a disease caused by repair deficits empowers you to maintain and rejuvenate your body at the cellular level. Since the introduction of the Beyond Health Model (One Disease—Two Causes—Six Pathways) in my first book, *Never Be Sick Again*, many thousands have used it to cure themselves of chronic illnesses and enjoy excellent health. I use the same concept here to show you how to eliminate the causes of cellular aging and help your body do the maintenance it is designed to do to keep you biologically young.

Accelerated aging is a mistake. The rate at which we age can be controlled. It is entirely possible to live a longer life and to greatly reduce the risk of age-related diseases—if you know the factors that accelerate aging and avoid them. By taking control of the aging process, you can reduce your biological age, delay aging, and enjoy a very long disease-free life. I invite you to learn how to do this.

CHAPTER 1

A New Outlook on Aging

You can't help getting older, but
you don't have to get old.

—Casey Stengel

The idea is to die young
as late as possible.

—Ashley Montagu

MOST PEOPLE BELIEVE THAT AGING IS something that just happens and that we have no control over it. What we typically call *aging*—changes in physical appearance, functionality of organs and tissues, disease, frailty, and senility—is a result of many factors. Changes at the genetic and cellular levels tip the balance between cellular damage and cellular repair. More damage and fewer repairs equal more aging and a progressive deterioration over time, making our bodies less viable and more vulnerable to disease.

Fortunately, it is possible to experience aging in an entirely different way than most people experience it. Mounting scientific evidence shows that *we can slow the aging process and live a long, healthy, vibrant life—free of disease and disability.* The purpose of this book is to remove the mystery, cut through the complexity, and make it all so simple that you will be in control of your health, the diseases you may develop, and *the rate at which you age.*

The rate at which you age and the diseases typically associated with old age are, for the most part, under your control. This is because *the rate at which you age is the direct result of the choices you make day in and day out throughout your lifetime.* Simple everyday choices, like what you buy at the grocery store, what you order at a restaurant, the personal care products you use, the stress you put on yourself, the radiation to which you expose yourself, and the amount of exercise and sleep you get can accelerate, slow down, or even reverse aging. It's time to rethink what being old is all about and what you can do about it. As it turns out, you can do a lot.

Modern Aging Is a Disease

Aging is a natural process and part of the human condition. *However, far from being a natural process, the accelerated aging that most of us are experiencing is a man-made disease and a mistake.* Despite all the scientific knowledge and technology that is available, our society has not learned how to achieve healthy aging. The purpose of this book is to teach you how to put to use what we already know so that you can add years of vital, healthy, and productive living to your lifespan.

In modern society, aging is a disease process. Poor diets, toxic exposures, stress, and lack of exercise all conspire to age a human body beyond its years. That's why aging, as most of us experience it, relates more to disease than chronology. This is good news, because we already know enough about disease to successfully intervene in the aging process. Good health slows down aging, causing one to look, feel, and actually be younger. To slow and even reverse aging, you must maintain or restore good health.

Think of two identical new cars in a dealer's lot. After a decade of use, the two cars can end up in vastly different conditions. One may still look and run like new, while the other is ready to be junked. How the cars have been driven and the care they have received makes all the difference. The same is true of your body. It rewards you with vibrant looks and excellent performance for correct use and maintenance, and it punishes you with breakdowns for failure to exercise proper maintenance. Cars more than a hundred years old can function like new if given proper maintenance—and so can you.

Your *chronological* age is the number of years since your birth. Your *biological* age is the way your body and mind function compared to average human experience, and it can measure less than or greater than your chronological age. Keep your body in good repair, and your biological age will stay significantly lower than your chronological age. That's the key to a long, vibrant, disease-free life. Of course you will still get old, but you will get old in the right way so you can remain active and strong, enjoying life to the fullest. As you begin to understand what keeps you biologically young, you will no longer fear the number of candles on your birthday cake. That's the promise I make to you in this book: to once and for all set chronological age apart from the aging symptoms and mortality associated with poor health. *I will show you why accelerated aging is an avoidable mistake and what you can do to stay biologically young.*

Evelyn's Story: A Choice to Stay Young

Evelyn died in 1997 at the age of 109. Evelyn lived a very spirited, high-quality life up until the last few weeks. She remained mentally sharp and physically active as an artist and a gardener. She grew most of her own food organically. Working in her flower and vegetable gardens, she got plenty of fresh air and sunshine along with a lot of exercise. Because she farmed organically, she was not exposed to toxic agricultural chemicals like other gardeners and farmers, and she ate her own fresh produce. Also, Evelyn didn't believe in doctors. She received no medical care—no drugs, no flu shots, nothing.

Let's think about what really set her apart from the average person. Did she come from an exceptionally hardy gene pool? No. Her exceptional health and longevity resulted from what she *did*, rather than what she was born with. The most important thing she did was to practice health-promoting habits and beliefs, and to make a choice to stay healthy and fit no matter what her age. In short, Evelyn ate high-quality fresh food; avoided toxins; got plenty of fresh air, exercise, and sunlight; and had a positive attitude toward life.

What Does a Fit 131 Look Like?

Consider the case of José Maria Roa, described by Morton Walker, DPM, in his 1985 book *Secrets of Long Life*. José and his family lived in a small village among a hardy group of people native to the Vilcabamba Valley, nestled in the Andes Mountains of Ecuador. At age 131, though his face was weatherworn, his mind was keen, his heart was healthy, his teeth were strong, and the lines around his face were born of smiles and the joy of a loving wife and family. Still working on his small hillside farm every day and enjoying an active sex life, José fathered his last child at the age of 107. When asked if he'd ever been sick, he replied, "Yes, I have been." José had had a few colds—that's it—in 131 years! José remained in excellent health until his death from old age at 137.

Was José an exception? Not at all. In his remote village, José's health and longevity were far from unusual—the average age at death was about 120. Dr. Walker asked if the older Vilcabambans suffered memory loss due to dementia. These long-lived people didn't understand the question because they had never experienced anything like dementia. In fact, they didn't even have words in their language to describe such a condition because it had never happened. Meanwhile, we are told that dementia is a disease of aging and the price we must pay for our so-called longevity. What nonsense!

José was not a medical miracle or an aberration of nature. This is what humans are capable of. It's just that we aren't doing what it takes to achieve it. People in Vilcabamba and in other areas around the world such as Hunza, Titicaca, Crete, the Caucasian Mountains, and Okinawa have all been known for their longevity. People in these societies rarely died before their 90s and commonly lived well into their 100s, reaching 120, 130, and older—free of disease. Today, residents of Okinawa have the world's highest life expectancy with the highest percentage of people living into their 100s in excellent health.

In March 1961, an article in the *Journal of the American Medical Association* reported on evidence that men in Hunza (in northeast Pakistan) lived to be 120 and even 140 years old. Hunza men and women older than 100 exhibited robust energy, in striking contrast to the fatigue in our society. These people lived simply and without doctors, hospitals, or nursing homes. In his 1968 book *Hunza,* J. M. Hoffman, PhD, who had spent years studying the people of the remote Hunza Valley in the Himalayas, quoted prominent physicians and scientists, including the presidents of the American Medical Association and the International Association of Gerontology, as saying that humans should live to be 120 to 150 years old. Estimates in biology journals project human life expectancy to exceed 135 years. Long life is our birthright. We should live to be at least 120, in vigorous health, maintaining physical and mental acuity. In the state of California, actuarial calculations show that average life expectancy for females would be 100 if only one type of disease were eliminated—heart disease—which is entirely preventable and reversible through diet and lifestyle. If eliminating one disease can do that, consider how much longer we might live by eliminating two or more of these so-called diseases.

Meanwhile, in our society, most of us are told—and usually believe—that illnesses such as cancer, arthritis, dementia, osteoporosis, diabetes, and heart disease are "diseases of aging." These chronic conditions are now epidemic, but they are not the inevitable result of growing older. Rather, they are the inevitable result of lifestyles that do not and cannot support human health.

Old Age Is No Longer What It Used to Be

In long-lived societies, when people died of old age, the typical death was sudden and rapid. Today, we mostly die of chronic diseases and death is slow and progressive, sometimes involving years of dependency and dysfunction. Very few people die of old age anymore. Instead, they are dying of completely preventable and curable chronic conditions that gradually overtake their bodies—all because they failed to provide their bodies the minimum support required for daily maintenance and repairs. *Today, there is abundant scientific evidence linking every one of the leading causes of death among the elderly to everyday lifestyle choices.*

Poor choices in diet and lifestyle affect our ability to make the energy that the body needs to be healthy. The more energy you can make, the healthier you are and the longer you will live. If you make less energy, you will have less ability to do cellular and DNA repair and to remove toxins from the body.

Let's take a look at the top six causes of death among adults sixty-five and older. All of these have been associated with lower energy production. In 2009, heart disease, cancer, chronic lower respiratory diseases, stroke, Alzheimer's disease, and diabetes made up 70 percent of all U.S. deaths. Most people believe that these diseases are a normal part of the aging process. *Wrong!* They are normal only to a society that eats a diet that is incapable of supplying the nutrition our bodies need to be healthy. Here's what we know about these diseases:

- **Heart disease.** Once a rare disease, this is the number-one cause of death in America. We are talking about heart failure, heart attack, and heart arrhythmia that can cause the heart to beat ineffectively and impair circulation. Numerous studies have linked heart disease to smoking, improper diet, exposure to toxins, and lack of exercise. Heart disease is almost always both preventable and reversible. We have created this epidemic; we can end it.

- **Cancer.** Cancer is the second-leading cause of death. Susceptibility to cancer rises with age. Yet, historically, cancer was a rare disease and virtually unknown among long-lived populations. We have created this epidemic by *diets, lifestyles, and environments* that promote cancer. Since we created it, we can un-create it. We know what causes cancer—a deficiency of oxygen respiration in our cells—and we know how to prevent and reverse it. There is no reason to have it. (See my book *Never Fear Cancer Again*.)

- **COPD.** Chronic obstructive pulmonary disease is an inflammatory disease typically involving chronic bronchitis or emphysema or both. COPD inhibits the lungs' ability to exchange carbon dioxide for oxygen. It makes breathing progressively harder, often making people feel like they are suffocating. Pulmonary diseases are often linked to environmental factors, such as a lifetime of smoking. They also result from a diet that is inadequate to protect and repair the lungs. Mostly self-inflicted, COPD is preventable.

- **Cerebrovascular disease.** Also known as *stroke*, cerebrovascular disease occurs when blood flow to a part of the brain stops because a blood vessel is either blocked (ischemic) or ruptured (hemorrhage). Deprived of blood and oxygen even for a few seconds, brain tissue can die, causing loss of mobility, hearing, speech, memory, and other vital functions. Almost all strokes can be prevented with a good diet and detoxification, and the disability from stroke can be mostly reversed by using techniques such as chelation therapy and hyperbaric oxygen.

- **Alzheimer's disease.** Alzheimer's is the most prevalent form of dementia, characterized by progressive memory loss, personality changes, and eventually a complete loss of function and ability. Alzheimer's deaths are increasing at alarming rates, and new statistics show that someone develops Alzheimer's every seventy-two seconds. In America, if you live into your eighties, your chances of suffering from significant mental decline are about

50 percent. But is this really a consequence of old age? Recall that in traditionally long-lived societies, conditions like Alzheimer's were completely unknown. Alzheimer's is just another epidemic we have created with poor diets, toxic exposures, and poor lifestyle choices. It is entirely preventable and even reversible, especially in its earlier stages, by making better choices.

- **Diabetes.** Type 2 diabetes, also known as *adult-onset diabetes,* is a chronic disease of elevated blood sugar due to insulin resistance. Diabetes increases the risk of stroke, heart disease, and other circulatory diseases. It also impairs immunity and causes multiple health problems, including slow wound healing and respiratory infections such as pneumonia. In fact, diabetes is the leading cause of blindness and of nontraumatic amputations. Here again is a disease that used to be rare and is now an epidemic. Type 2 diabetes is entirely preventable and easily reversible with proper diet, supplements, and exercise. There is no reason for anyone to have it, yet about 25 million Americans have Type 2 diabetes.

As you see, our leading medical problems are preventable and even reversible. Even though it has been obscured from the general public, the knowledge is there to vastly improve the way we age. Why not take advantage of it? When asked about how they want to live and die, most people say they want to live a long and vigorous life and then to die quickly, at an advanced age, with little suffering. This is the way it should be, and almost everyone is capable of achieving this goal. When functioning as intended, the human body is capable of repairing extensive damage and living well beyond a hundred years. Standing in our way are the human-made diseases that rob us of a *true* old-age experience. What's more, these diseases are beginning to threaten both our health and our wealth at younger ages. Our high rates of disease will continue until we stop believing that disease is a random event that can happen to anyone. To the contrary, health is a duty. We need to take responsibility for our health, and use the knowledge we already have to prevent and reverse disease.

Aging Crisis Strikes All Ages

Accelerated aging is now an out-of-control epidemic, and it is even affecting our young. *Our young people are old!* So-called diseases of old age are no longer limited to the elderly. Children are being diagnosed with hypertension (high blood pressure), adult diabetes, and cancer. In fact, after accidents, cancer is the leading cause of death for children and those in their twenties and thirties. Nearly half of all deaths from eight categories of cancer, including bone, cervix, and thyroid, occur in those under thirty-four. New cases of "adult" diabetes in children are skyrocketing. Our young people are so old and sick, they are going to add an unbearable burden to a health care system that is already in serious trouble. Having achieved enormous advances in science and medicine, why are we experiencing the largest epidemic of chronic disease in human history?

The problem with aging is not that we have no choice in the matter, but that, *since the time we are born, we are conditioned to make poor choices.* Processed foods, sedentary lifestyles, toxic household products, stressful daily routines, and invasive medical treatments are all adding up to advance the onset of chronic illness and accelerate our aging. As individuals, and as a society, we are paying the price with a full-scale aging crisis.

What Does Premature Aging Look Like?

Strokes are our fourth-leading cause of death, and most strokes occur in the elderly. But here's a surprise: our young people are having more strokes today than they did just a decade ago. A 2011 study in the *Annals of Neurology* found that the youngest group of ischemic (blood clot) stroke patients—fifteen- to thirty-four-year-olds—experienced 30 percent more strokes in 2008 than they did in 1995. The increase among the thirty-five- to forty-four-year-olds was 37 percent.

Just as it's possible to make yourself younger when you are in your nineties, it's also possible to make yourself older in the prime of your life. Unfortunately, more and more people are doing just that. How? Hypertension (high blood pressure) and obesity are risk factors for stroke. More than half of the young people in the ischemic stroke study had hypertension. Unheard of in the past, teen hypertension has become a fact, and the main driver is obesity. According to the American Obesity Association, 30 percent of American teens are overweight and 15 percent are obese. That's triple what these rates were in 1980. Compounding the problem, fat cells produce a flood of health-damaging free radicals that accelerate the aging process.

Besides being overweight, our teens and young adults have too much stress and caffeine and not enough sleep, all risk factors for hypertension, stroke, and aging. Add to this too much sugar, too few essential fatty acids, the wrong pH, and vitamin and mineral deficiencies, and you have a recipe for rapid aging—no matter what your age.

Increasing Life Expectancy Is a Myth

How long can people expect to live? There is no fixed theoretical limit. But some clarity is in order. The impression that human life span is increasing is mostly a myth. We are confusing *maximum* human life span with *average* life expectancy. The numbers usually quoted are the *average* of all deaths, including infant mortality. Average life expectancy has been steadily increasing mainly because fewer babies are dying. In fact, *the increase in average life expectancy is almost entirely due to decreasing infant mortality.*

In 1907, the average life expectancy for a male in the United States was forty-five; it is now seventy-five. Were men really dying at forty-five? Not exactly. In the early 1900s more than 50 percent of all deaths involved children under age fourteen, bringing the average down to forty-five years. By 2001, only 1.6 percent of the total deaths occurred among the young, bringing the average up. Likewise, the average life expectancy for men in ancient Greece was forty. Yet the ancient Greek philosophers typically lived over the age of ninety. It is the inclusion of infant and child mortality in calculating life expectancy that is creating the mistaken impression that, historically, adults died young and that life expectancy for all ages is now greater than ever. The truth is that the maximum human life span hasn't changed much for thousands of years. Moses died at age 120, Egyptian pharaoh Ramses II at age 90, Michelangelo at 89, King George III at 81, and Benjamin Franklin at 84. Hosius of Córdoba, the man who convinced Constantine the Great to call the First Council of Nicaea, lived to age 102. Are we living longer?

The point is that today more children make it into adulthood. Infant mortality has decreased dramatically because of a lack of famine, good sewer systems, safe water supplies, less crowded living conditions, and modern medicine's ability to treat accident victims successfully. However, when we look at older adults, the picture is far less reassuring. In 1850, a seventy-year-old white American male could expect to survive for ten more years. In 2003, the average life expectancy of a seventy-year-old white male was thirteen years. That's only a three-year gain over the course of 153 years, despite enormous advances in science and technology. Then consider that those extra three years are not healthy ones. We may be living a few years longer, but are we living better? On key measures of health, Americans are falling behind other developed nations, and the number of years of living with a chronic disease continues to increase for the average American. We are living a little longer, but we spend that time struggling with chronic illness and running up steeply rising, *budget-busting* costs.

Americans, in particular, are doing a terrible job at extending adult life span. According to the Average Life Expectancy Chart published in a 2009 article on *Disabled World*, the average American dies at age seventy-eight. While most Americans think this is really good, it's not. This puts American life expectancy at thirty-eighth in the world, behind even Cuba, Costa Rica, and Chile. This is down from twenty-fourth in 1999 and fifth place in 1950. If anything, Americans are going backward. Even though we spend more on health care than any nation on Earth, the World Health Organization ranks us only thirty-seventh in the world in overall health. Our health care spending has increased, but our health and life expectancy have not, and are projected to sharply decline in the coming decades due to the poor health of our children. By any measurement of performance, Americans have the most ineffective health care system in the developed world—spending much more and getting much less.

We Can No Longer Afford Premature Aging

Did you know that 45 percent of the U.S. federal budget goes for Medicare, Medicaid, and Social Security benefits? According to the Congressional Budget Office, if no changes are made, these costs will amount to 54 percent by 2022, and covering them will require a considerable increase in taxes or government borrowing, or cuts in other programs. As this country's 77 million baby boomers age and health care costs continue to skyrocket, the government's ability to pay for these programs becomes increasingly difficult and perhaps even impossible.

The single most important factor driving rapidly rising health care costs is our epidemic of chronic and degenerative disease. We must eliminate this epidemic before it bankrupts our governments and businesses. Unfortunately, conventional medicine is clueless on how to stop this epidemic. We must find better ways to address these problems, based on cutting-edge science and common sense.

Anti-Aging Industry Is a Sea of Misinformation

If we haven't found the elixir of youth yet, it hasn't been for the lack of trying. For the last decade, the U.S. demand for anti-aging products has been rising by almost 10 percent annually. Compare this with only 1.6 percent per year average economic (GDP) growth for the same period, and you get the picture: Americans are worried about aging. An ever-increasing portion of our income goes toward our hopes of staying young. Demand for memory improvement, vision care, and prostate care products are growing the fastest. Other top spending categories are bone and joint care, sexual dysfunction and impotence, menopause, aging skin care, and hair loss. Spending on anti-aging products by Americans was $80 billion in 2011 and is projected to reach $114 billion by 2015.

While new aging interventions are arriving almost daily, there is very little science behind these products. Good science is expensive, time-consuming, and often inconclusive. By contrast, talk is cheap, fast, and contagious. Plus, there are few restrictions on claims that manufacturers can make for advertising purposes. Where most anti-aging products are concerned, consumers are on their own, paying $10,000 or more for a facelift, $15,000 per year for human growth hormone treatment, and $18,000 per year for high-end skincare products.

The sellers are not in the market to make you younger. They are in the market to make money. The National Institute on Aging advises consumers to be skeptical about purported anti-aging products and procedures. The institute maintains that, to date, no treatment has been proven to slow or reverse the aging process, and many have been found harmful or ineffective. Take, for example, hormone replacement therapies.

As we age, the body slows down its production of certain hormones that affect our fertility, sexual function, mood, energy, and physical appearance. Can we fix this problem by replacing the body's own hormones with manufactured ones? The industry touts synthetic, "bioidentical" and "individualized" hormone replacement drugs as a cure for aging. However, no study to date has credited hormone drugs with significant anti-aging benefits. On the contrary, studies clearly show a link between estrogen replacement and breast cancer in women. The National Institutes of Health warn that hormone replacement therapy increases the risk of cancer, heart disease, and stroke. A good reason to be wary of hormone treatments is that the human endocrine system is simply too complicated. There are about fifty known hormones, every one of them interacting with every other hormone in the body. When you artificially increase the supply of one hormone, you can unbalance the function of all the others.

Most skincare products are notoriously useless and generally toxic, ironically more so for older women, whose bodies are already suffering from toxic overload (more on this in Chapter 5, "The Toxin Pathway"). The September 2011 *Consumer Reports* tested several brands of over-the-counter facial serums, wrinkle creams, and eye creams. The tests revealed that even the best performers reduced the average depth of the wrinkles by less than 10 percent, a change almost invisible to the naked eye.

The upshot is that there is no evidence that any of the anti-aging regimens on the market today can successfully intervene in the natural aging process. The good news is that in order to age well, all we need to do is to allow the body to function naturally and shut down the disease processes that result in accelerated aging. The advice you've heard all along—eat a healthy diet, exercise regularly, and don't smoke—is correct, but incomplete and deceptively simple. In order to benefit from it, you need to know what a healthy diet is for you, how exercise fits into your lifestyle, and all the rest of the important but overlooked factors in your environment that affect your health. Most importantly, you need to understand what is behind accelerated aging in our culture and why you are likely to be aging prematurely right now. When you understand this clearly, I promise you, you will feel differently about your future. Making healthy choices and staying biologically young will become a way of life. The search for a miracle cure is over.

What Is Aging?

We attribute our decline to "aging" when we can't think of any other reason we are "going downhill." Yet passage of time alone does not explain what happens to our bodies. Nor does it account for vast differences in rates and modes of aging among individuals.

Aging can be measured in a variety of ways, including hormone levels, plasma proteins, glycation of collagen, DNA unwinding rate, proliferative capacity of fibroblast-like cells, T-cell subset values, skin elasticity, lung capacity, maximum oxygen uptake, the amount of thiobarbituric acid-reactive substances (TBARS) in the blood, and telomere shortening. Wow! That's a long list. But have no fear; I am going to simplify it for you.

Aging affects the entire body, which is completely interconnected. As science discovers new links in the pathways of aging, new products will pour into the market, claiming to fix one measure of aging or another, similar to today's wrinkle creams and hormone replacement therapies. Targeting the outward or even inward symptoms of aging, like collagen in your skin, hormone levels in your blood, or the DNA in your cells—without addressing the cause—will only waste your money and expose you to dangerous side effects. A better approach is to eliminate the root cause of premature aging, and then all the symptoms will improve at the same time. That's what I'll show you how to do.

Aging and Inflammation

One way to account for the differences in rates and modes of aging among individuals is inflammation. Inflammation is one of the common denominators of disease. *Every* chronic disease is an inflammatory disease. No matter what so-called disease you have, from cancer to heart disease, or accelerated aging, inflammation is a major part of your problem. Learning how to prevent and reverse inflammation will go a long way toward preventing and reversing almost all disease, as well as slowing the aging process and helping you to stay biologically young and vigorous for a lifetime.

What is inflammation? It is an essential defense mechanism that serves as an all-purpose protection against invaders and trauma. It is the body's natural and healthy response to injury, irritation, or infection. If you cut your finger, the body immediately begins an inflammatory process that neutralizes harmful microorganisms, helps to repair the wound, and cleans up the debris resulting from the injury. *Temporary* inflammation is beneficial when needed, but *chronic* inflammation is disastrous. When inflammation is turned on and never turned off, it generates a constant supply of free radicals that overwhelm your antioxidant defenses and damage DNA, aging you and causing disease of every description. For example, most hip replacements originate with inflammatory damage to the joint. A better idea is to protect the joint from inflammation and keep it in good repair; then it will last a lifetime. The amount of inflammation in your body is a powerful predictor of aging, age-related disease, and whether or not you will become fragile in old age.

In an interview with *Discover* magazine, Russell Tracy, professor of pathology and biochemistry at the University of Vermont College of Medicine, stated, "Inflammatory factors predict virtually all bad outcomes in humans." For example, one reason we lose lean muscle mass as we age is because inflammation breaks down skeletal muscle. Osteoporosis, declining lung function, and old-age depression can all be triggered by inflammation. In diabetes, inflammation and insulin resistance track together, while in Alzheimer's patients, senility-associated amyloid plaques build up in areas of the brain where there are lots of inflammatory cells and cytokines (cytokines are inflammation producing proteins). Research shows that inflammatory activity blocks memory formation. Inflammation also contributes to the shortening of telomeres, because it prompts faster turnover of cells in the immune system and other tissues.

The key to longevity is to avoid chronic inflammation. Unfortunately, chronic systemic inflammation is epidemic. Why is this happening? It's happening because we eat a diet and live in an environment that promotes inflammation. Our diet is rich in pro-inflammatory factors, while lacking antioxidants and other nutrients that help to prevent and control inflammation. Being overweight makes things worse, because fat cells spur more inflammation, making aging and chronic diseases strike earlier. Dietary restriction is one way to inhibit the inflammatory response, which explains why low-calorie diets promote longevity. Dietary restriction also reduces insulin resistance and slows the onset and progression of dementia. In Chapters 3 and 4, I will tell you more about how to control inflammation through your diet.

Understanding Telomeres

Inflammation shortens telomeres, and shortened telomeres shorten your life. Telomeres are DNA caps at the end of chromosomes that act like shoelace tips to keep the chromosome from unraveling. Every time a cell divides, some of the telomere length is lost. Eventually, enough is lost that the chromosome unravels and the cell dies. Research shows that telomere shortening is part of the aging process—a biological marker of aging. The shorter your telomeres, the higher your risk of dying. Factors such as chronic inflammation speed up telomere shortening, while certain nutrients help to repair telomeres and keep them long. You will learn more about how to prevent telomere shortening in Chapter 4.

Aging Is Repair Deficits

Aging is not unique to humans—or to living organisms. Cars age. How do you keep a car in good condition? You change the oil. You top off fluids. You rotate tires. You replace brake pads. In other words, you do what is called *maintenance*. If you keep your car in good repair, it will continue to work well and look like new. The human body works the same way. If you support the body's normal repair process, it will serve you well for more than a century. In order to fix your car, you need the correct replacement parts, tools, and instruction manuals. For example, if you put the wrong oil in a car, you will damage the engine. We humans need the correct oil, too. While most of us know better than to put the wrong oil in our car, we consistently put the wrong oils in our bodies with devastating results. What you put in your body becomes the raw material for building your cells. The body makes more than 10 million new cells every second. If you use high-quality building materials to make those cells, and if you assemble them according to the correct blueprint, then every new cell will operate properly, keeping you healthy and biologically young. If not, you get the opposite results, and that is what's happening. Junk in, junk out! Our junk-food diets and toxic exposures are crippling our ability to do normal preventive maintenance, and then we wonder why even our children are old.

What people refer to as aging is really the accumulation of repair deficits. Your body is a self-repairing system, and many of these repairs take place during sleep. One reason most of us wake up every morning with repair deficits is that we are not getting enough sleep. Think about it. We start every day with our maintenance overdue and our repairs for yesterday's wear and tear unfinished. By the end of the day, more maintenance comes due and more repair work is required. If you keep putting off maintenance and repairs on your car, eventually your car will break down. A body that is not repaired daily builds up damage until it no longer functions as intended—then people rush off to their doctor for drugs, surgery, and artificial replacement parts. We accept all this as normal and never stop to think about what we are doing wrong.

A body malfunctions when a large number of cells malfunction. There are two causes of cellular malfunction: *deficiency* and *toxicity*. Deficiency results in a lack of repair materials, and toxicity scrambles the blueprints and disables repair machinery. Prevent deficiency and toxicity—give the body the raw materials it needs to do the repairs and keep the repair machinery operating smoothly—and the body will remain in good repair and be healthy. Each cell carries within itself its own instruction manual—the DNA. We already have all the necessary maintenance manuals and tools (the metabolic machinery) to carry out daily repairs. *All you need to do is supply adequate nutrients and also avoid toxins to keep the repair machinery from malfunctioning.*

You can control deficiency and toxicity through the Six Pathways to health or disease: Nutrition, Toxin, Mental, Physical, Genetic, and Medical. I will discuss each pathway in detail, showing you the steps others have taken, and you can take today, to eliminate repair deficits in your body. What this means to you is the opportunity to live a very long, healthy, and productive life, free of disease and the need for others to care for you. To age successfully, all you have to do is take advantage of the scientific knowledge backed by many years of research, and stop the destructive practices that, unfortunately, have become entrenched in our culture.

Keep a car in good repair and it will age gracefully and continue to give good service. It is the same with your body. If you make consistent, high-quality repairs to your body, you will never wear out your parts. In short, nobody needs a pacemaker, a knee or a hip replacement, or any other replacement. People can start this maintenance process at any age and still get benefits. It's amazing how much aging can be reversed if you improve your diet, minimize toxins, and shift your body into repair mode, allowing it to do the repairs that it is already programmed to do. The more damage you have done to your car, the more effort and time it will take to repair it, but it can be done. Yet nothing good will happen until you start the repair process. *As I discuss the Six Pathways, I urge you to focus on the concrete steps you can take within each pathway to limit damage, promote repairs, and prevent repair deficits. This is the secret to graceful aging.*

The Bottom Line ———————————————

✓ We can't avoid aging, but today aging has become associated with disease, dysfunction, disability, and dependency. Although this kind of accelerated aging has become accepted as normal, it is not natural and is almost entirely related to our unnatural lifestyles.

✓ Most people want to live a long and vigorous life, and then to die quickly with little suffering at an old age. This is how it should be, and what most people are capable of doing.

✓ By working with nature, instead of against it, and making different lifestyle choices, we can control how we age.

✓ To keep a car in good condition over a long period of time, you need to maintain it. It is the same with the human body, except that, unlike your car, the body is a self-repairing, self-maintaining system.

✓ The body cannot make needed repairs and replacement parts unless we supply it with the nutrients it needs and prevent toxins from interfering with the repair machinery.

✓ When repair deficits accumulate, aging occurs.

✓ This book will teach you how to limit damage, promote repairs, and prevent repair deficits. This is the secret to graceful, healthy aging.

CHAPTER 2

What Is Disease?

Health is a state of complete physical,
mental, and social well-being and not merely
the absence of disease or infirmity.
—Preamble to the Constitution of the World Health Organization

Whatever a cell does has to be paid for—
and the currency of living systems, with
which the cell has to pay, is energy.
—Nobel laureate Albert V. Szent-György, MD, PhD

I F WE COULD CONCEIVE OF A ROBUST OLD AGE, free of disease
and disability, we would not dread getting old. It is the prospect
of having to suffer the indignity of a feeble mind and a malfunctioning body that most of us fear. In our culture, we have accepted

the belief that we have little control over aging, and that senility and frailty are natural and inevitable consequences of advancing years. But this is not true. The accelerated aging that is so prevalent in modern societies is a disease, and it is caused by accumulated repair deficits and a breakdown in our energy production and storage systems. Here's what you need to know about disease: when correctly understood at the cellular and molecular level, *almost all disease can be prevented and reversed*, and that includes the disease and disability that accompany premature aging.

There Is Only One Disease

To solve any problem, it helps to understand its causes. This is why to prevent or cure disease—and slow the aging process—you need to understand what disease is and what causes it. Once you understand the causes, you can do something about them, but two conditions are necessary: (1) you must be willing to make changes; and (2) you must know which changes to make. The scientific knowledge we already have is sufficient to slow the aging process and even reverse biological age—we have only to put it to use. Multiple scientific experiments and the experiences of many individuals have demonstrated this point. To help you put this knowledge to use, let me simplify how to think about the body and its diseases.

How is this for simplicity? *There is only one disease!* Not thousands of diseases, as we are used to thinking. What is this one disease? Malfunctioning cells. Our bodies are made of tens of trillions of microscopic units of life called cells. Each of us starts life as a single cell in our mother. That one cell eventually grows into a vast community of cells that communicate and cooperate with each other, forming a single organism that functions as who we are. All tissues and organs are made of cells. All bodily functions are carried out by cells, and cells are specialized according to the function they perform.

Disease originates inside of cells. If all of your individual cells are functioning normally, then all of your cells can communicate with one another, and your body is self-regulating, self-repairing, and balanced. When your body is in balance, you are healthy and you *cannot* be sick. This balanced state is called *homeostasis*.

When you are in homeostasis, your body regulates its internal conditions, regardless of external conditions. A simple example of homeostasis is the body's ability to regulate and maintain its internal temperature within a narrow range in both hot and cold weather. If your temperature gets too low or too high, you will die, and it is the same for many other factors that need to be regulated. When cells malfunction, the body's ability to produce energy, communicate, self-regulate, and self-repair is damaged. In a typical day, we put a lot of wear and tear on the body. If your body is not fully self-repairing daily, you will develop repair deficits, and your body will soon let you know. Any illness is a sign that you need repairs that your body isn't making. Repair deficits manifest as aging, disease, and disability. In fact, all chronic disease involves repair deficits. This is why chronic diseases are degenerative—getting worse as you age. If we do nothing about them, the repair deficits can only grow larger with the passage of time. Whatever disease label your physician has pasted on you, whether it's allergies, arthritis, diabetes, cancer, Alzheimer's, or osteoporosis, all are due to cellular malfunction and repair deficits.

Infirmity and disease cannot happen unless cells malfunction. Alzheimer's disease is cells malfunctioning in the memory part of the brain. Parkinson's disease is cells malfunctioning in the motor part of the brain. Macular degeneration is cells malfunctioning in the eye. However, any localized health problem is a sign of cellular malfunction throughout the body. Symptoms may be most pronounced in one particular part of the body, but they are evidence of a breakdown of cellular function and the loss of homeostatic balance throughout the body. To think of specific disorders as different diseases is self-defeating because it obscures the true nature of disease. All so-called diseases are merely symptoms of the one disease—cellular malfunction. To empower yourself to prevent and reverse age-related illnesses, you need to focus on what is common to all disease, not what's different about each case. *No matter what the symptoms, when you restore cells to normal function, you are cured, and the symptoms go away.* Keeping things simple, you don't need to concern yourself with trillions of cells. If you learn how to make one cell work right, you can make them all work right.

The Two Causes of Aging and Disease

As you have just learned, there is only one disease: cellular malfunction. To stay healthy and biologically young, you must prevent or eliminate what is causing this disease. *There are only two causes of cellular malfunction: deficiency and toxicity.* Either cells are getting *too little* of what they need or *too much* of what they don't need. The number of days we are on this earth does not destroy our health and age us. Deficiency, toxicity, and the resulting repair deficits do.

You might ask, how can deficiency and toxicity be the cause of all disease? Doesn't stress cause disease? It sure does, but through the same two causes: deficiency and toxicity. During stressful times, the body produces stress chemicals, such as the hormone cortisone, and releases them into the bloodstream. Chronic stress causes a buildup of stress chemicals in the body, which has a toxic effect. Manufacturing stress chemicals depletes the body of critical nutrients, causing deficiency. Even infectious and genetic diseases manifest because of deficiency and toxicity. For example, a bacterial infection can kill you because of deadly toxins produced by the bacteria. When genes malfunction, they cause either deficiency or toxicity, or both. In every case you might think of, it always comes back to deficiency and toxicity—the two causes that are common to all disease.

Think of each cell in your body as a vast industrial park containing thousands of factories, producing tens of thousands of life-sustaining chemicals every day. Some of these chemicals are hormones to help regulate your body; neurotransmitters to enable you to learn, think, and remember; and antibodies to keep you free of infection. Each cell contains hundreds of powerhouses called mitochondria to produce the energy of life. There are also warehouses, traffic directors, communication systems, nutrient delivery systems, waste disposal systems, security systems, a central computer, and much more. All of this metabolic machinery knows how to function perfectly when the right raw materials (nutrients) are available and toxic substances are not interfering with normal operations.

If even one nutrient is chronically lacking, your body will not be able to make enough of the right chemicals. In each cell, there are about 100,000 chemical reactions taking place every second, accompanied by literally trillions of individual activities. Our job is to support all of this. When we don't, we age and get sick. *A chronic deficiency of even one nutrient will create repair deficits, make us sick, and age us faster.* This is why it is so significant that the average American is chronically deficient in at least several essential nutrients. We also know that even one toxin can disable critical metabolic pathways or give incorrect instructions to the cells, creating chaos in the cells and the body. Even worse, studies show that combinations of toxins acting together can be thousands of times more damaging than any one toxin acting alone. Meanwhile, the average American is a toxic dumpsite, accumulating an overload of hundreds of different toxins in our body tissues.

Sarah's Story: Aging in Reverse

Sarah is the mother of a friend. A bright and capable woman, Sarah had been very active her whole life. In addition to pursuing a challenging career and raising a family, she used to volunteer at local charities and was elected to her town's school committee. When she was in her early sixties, Sarah's health began to decline. First, she was diagnosed with high blood pressure and then high cholesterol. Her doctor prescribed medications, but these made her dizzy and gave her headaches. Additional prescriptions followed to counteract the effects of the drugs she was already taking. In the meantime, Sarah was falling apart. When I met her, she was no longer the "Committee Sarah" everyone knew. She had arthritis, was light-headed, and chronically fatigued. She suffered short-term memory loss and would easily get lost. My friend was dismayed at his mother's rapid decline and asked if I could help her. At first, Sarah wouldn't hear of it. To her, her doctor was God, and what did I know? When Sarah finally agreed to talk to me, I recommended that she stop consuming what I call the Big Four (sugar, wheat, processed oils, and dairy), add more organic fresh fruits and vegetables to her diet, and get on a high-quality supplement program. I looked at sources of toxins and recommended different brands of toothpaste, shampoo, and household cleaning products. I also suggested that she get off the nine prescription drugs she was taking. This was a hard sell, but eventually she acquiesced and got off the drugs. This substantially reduced her toxic load, and she began making improvements. Now in her seventies, she is looking and feeling fabulous. Sarah has all the spark and vigor of her younger years. She had never imagined it was possible to grow younger until she gave it a try.

What Your Doctor Will Not Tell You

How is it possible that a few simple changes to diet and lifestyle can restore youth and cure disease, while the medical establishment fumbles, achieving meager results at great expense? The shocking truth is that today's conventional medicine is not based on solid science.

Conventional Medicine Fails to Meet the Challenge of Chronic Disease

When it comes to intervening in crisis situations, such as treating traumatic injuries, conventional medicine shines; in the United States we enjoy the best emergency room medicine in the world. But with chronic diseases, like cancer, heart disease, arthritis, or diabetes, conventional medicine comes up woefully short. Far from effecting cures, the best it has to offer is *cut and drug therapies*— removing ailing body parts with surgery and subduing symptoms with toxic medications. These medications interfere with normal body chemistry, causing even more disease.

Although it pays lip service to prevention, typical medical testing doesn't identify problems until they are already far advanced. One of the most frustrating and yet one of the most common occurrences in doctors' offices today is this: A patient comes in complaining of fatigue, nausea, sinus congestion, skin problems, or any of a number of bothersome symptoms, and the doctor orders an expensive battery of tests. When all the test results come back, the patient is often told that "nothing is wrong." But something has to be wrong or the patient would not be experiencing these symptoms.

The fact is that conventional medical testing will not diagnose you with a specific disease until you are already very sick. Health exists along a continuum, with *perfect health* at one end and *death* at the other. By the time conventional medicine can diagnose you with one of their so-called diseases, your health is already closer to the death end of the continuum than it is to perfect health.

By the time conventional tests allow a diagnosis, "heroic" measures such as drugging or cutting are often considered necessary, while lifestyle improvements and supplements are considered inadequate. For patients, fear enters into the equation, which tends to make them much more compliant and willing to obey their doctor's orders. A more sophisticated and much sounder approach—taken by some alternative and functional-medicine health practitioners— is to find dysfunction and imbalance much earlier, so that interventions can be made sooner along the continuum. Such interventions are usually based on the so-called softer therapies, such as lifestyle improvements, herbs, and supplements, which focus on improving and normalizing function rather than suppressing symptoms. These healers often choose to work with patients as partners and support a patient's desire to be proactive in improving their health.

To cure a disease, or to reverse a disease process, you must address its cause(s). Disease is not caused by having body parts you don't need or by pharmaceutical drug deficiencies. There are only two causes of disease: nutrient deficiency and toxicity.

The human body is a miraculous and extremely complex system that took over a billion years to design. Between 50 and 100 trillion cells in the body are in continuous communication with one another through a vast network of physical, chemical, and electro-magnetic pathways—it staggers the imagination. Trying to manipulate these biochemical pathways with drugs to suppress symptoms in such a complex and interactive system is an act of lunacy that is doomed to failure. Why not simply support this miraculous body by giving it what it needs and protecting it from harm? It will then do what it is designed to do and regulate itself. What a concept!

Laura's Story: Never Be the Same Doctor Again

After running a busy internal medicine practice for twenty years, Laura was depressed, disillusioned, and about to quit medicine. Laura had chosen to go to medical school so that she could relieve pain and suffering and help people live better lives. But in the middle of her career, she came to an astounding conclusion: "I have just spent twenty years doing harm instead of good."

After my first book, *Never Be Sick Again*, was published, I received literally thousands of responses. People wrote saying that they had been able to cure themselves of chronic health problems after their doctors had completely failed. Among these was a letter from Laura. Laura was trained in conventional medicine and, after twenty years of practice, had come to realize that what she had learned about disease in medical school was fundamentally wrong, and that the drugs and vaccines she had prescribed for the last twenty years had harmed her patients. She was disillusioned and depressed and had decided to quit medicine. "Thank you for changing my life," she wrote. "After I read your book, I decided to stay in medicine, but to practice it the way you suggest. Since then, I have been able to help hundreds of patients and I have rediscovered meaning and purpose in my work."

Once Laura understood what disease is and why it happens, she saw that eliminating deficiency and toxicity, and restoring cells to normal function, was the only sensible way to practice medicine. What has helped Laura's patients and many of our readers more than anything else is realizing that they have the power to create health and well-being in their lives. Conventional medicine believes there are thousands of diseases and it keeps inventing new ones. This disempowers individuals. Can any one person understand thousands of diseases? This is why patients are often referred to any number of specialized experts, and even *they* don't understand it all. Notice what happens at this point: *nobody is responsible for your health*! This is because no one, including you, has the whole picture. All of this changes when you understand there is only one disease with two causes.

Repair Your Cells

The way we define a problem and the way we go about fixing it are intimately related. If you say, "I have arthritis," then you want to find an arthritis specialist who can treat your arthritis for you. Notice the word *arthritis* doesn't explain what is happening to your body. It doesn't tell you how you got it and doesn't empower you to cure it. Indeed, it does the opposite. It makes you feel way out of your league and forces you to run to the medical establishment for help. Why? Because they have a cure? No! Because they invented the word *arthritis*—which makes them sound as if they know something that you don't. Likewise, if you say, "I am aging" or "I've aged," you are implicitly blaming the passage of time. So that's that: you can't stop the clock or erase the past, and the future looks bleak. *If, on the other hand, you define your problem as lack of cellular repair, due to deficiency and toxicity, then the solution is clear: repair your cells!*

This may sound ridiculous at first. How do I repair my own cells? Think back to my car analogy. To repair a car you need spare parts, tools, and a manual. Your local repair shop will have the repair manuals and the tools. The parts come from elsewhere. Likewise, your cells come equipped with tools and instructions to repair and replicate themselves. The spare parts come from your diet. Your cells already know how to fix themselves. *The body's ability to self-repair is one of the most fundamental principles of health and life itself.* All you need to do is supply the raw materials and make sure the repair machinery doesn't get disabled by toxins. *Change the conditions in your body from those that favor aging and disease to those that favor health and repair, and grow younger.*

You don't need to be good at science, nor do you have to know all there is to know about cells, as long as what you do know is sufficient to keep them in good repair. This book will provide you with the necessary knowledge, not only to reverse disease, but also to turn back the clock to a younger you. Read on.

An Example of One Disease

Consider the case of Alex, a computer programmer from San Francisco. Alex went to see his physician, complaining of asthma, arthritis pain, and depression. After a thorough examination, his doctor also diagnosed him with osteoporosis and high blood pressure. According to conventional medicine's view of disease, Alex was suffering from five diagnosable diseases. His doctor prescribed a beta-blocker for his blood pressure and a non-steroidal anti-inflammatory drug for his arthritis. He then referred Alex to a pulmonary specialist for his asthma, a psychiatrist for his depression, and a bone specialist for his osteoporosis. These specialists put Alex on a number of additional drugs: a bronchodilator and a corticosteroid for his asthma, Zoloft for his depression, and Fosamax for his osteoporosis. None of these drugs will cure anything. All they do is suppress symptoms. Not surprisingly, the combination of these toxic chemicals made Alex even sicker. When he complained to his doctor again, his doctor wrote new prescriptions to suppress the side effects of the old ones. The more drugs Alex took, the sicker he got.

Had Alex's physicians known what you now know, that there is only one disease, it would have been a different story. Alex's conventionally trained physicians treated him for what they thought were five different diseases. Wrong! There is only one disease: malfunctioning cells caused by deficiency and toxicity. When Alex asked for my advice, I explained why there is only one disease and advised him to look for why his cells were malfunctioning. After doing a heavy metals challenge test, it was discovered that Alex's cells were malfunctioning because they were toxic with too much mercury. Even at extremely low concentrations, mercury can cause all of the so-called diseases that Alex was experiencing. In addition, mercury toxicity causes many deficiencies by disabling critical enzymes. Alex had many mercury fillings in his mouth, and he frequently ate mercury-containing fish. To rid his body of mercury, Alex had his amalgam fillings replaced, eliminated fish from his diet, and underwent a medical procedure called intravenous chelation. He improved his diet by adding more fresh fruits and vegetables and took high-quality supplements to detoxify and rebuild his system. By eliminating deficiency and toxicity and restoring his cells to normal function, Alex was cured of all his so-called diseases. Had he not done this, he would have remained on toxic prescription drugs for the rest of his life, getting sicker and sicker with each passing year. Once you understand there is only one disease, curing almost any so-called disease becomes possible.

Your Health Is a Continuum

As I said before, the state of your health is not merely a presence or absence of certain diseases. Your health is a continuum of conditions from perfect homeostasis on one end to terminal illness on the other. Homeostasis is the only stable health condition. Whenever cells have started to malfunction anywhere in your body, you can go in one of two directions: either toward better health or toward more disease. In Alex's case, with multiple prescription drugs adding to his toxic overload, he was clearly moving full-speed toward aging and disease, until he correctly addressed the cause of his symptoms. Similarly, in our society, virtually all of us—whether we have serious complaints or not—are somewhere in between perfect health and death. As such, there are steps we can take to help move the body toward health. But how do we know what is happening on the cellular level, when everything seems to be okay on the surface?

Most people think going to their doctor for checkups will keep them in good health. While monitoring your health is important, as we saw from Alex's example, a conventional doctor most likely won't help you in the early stages of cellular malfunction, precisely when the imbalance is the easiest to correct. Moreover, when the tests finally indicate that something is wrong, the usual response is prescribing medications that merely suppress the symptoms, while actually adding to the deficiency and toxicity already present in the body. What can you do to monitor your own health? Here's an idea . . .

pH and Your Health

Wouldn't it be convenient if we could measure the state of our health using a single number? Unfortunately, such a number doesn't exist. However, there is a number that is extremely useful.

That number is the pH, or acid-alkaline balance, of your cells. Fortunately, this number is easy for you to measure, and it is also entirely under your control. Diet affects pH, which in turn goes a long way toward controlling your health and the rate at which you age. A slightly alkaline pH is best, so it's worth making the effort to eat an alkaline diet.

You may have read or heard the expression "alkalize or die." Perhaps you have wondered if that is valid, or even what it means. Here is why pH is so important to your health and longevity: pH is a measure of the acidity or alkalinity of a solution. Aqueous solutions with a pH less than 7 are acidic (think vinegar), 7 is defined as neutral (like water), and greater than 7 is alkaline (think lye). The pH of your cells and body fluids has a major effect on your health. How major? If your pH is wrong, *nothing* will be right!

To function normally and keep your body in homeostasis, your cells need a proper environment. This means that numerous factors, including temperature, glucose levels, oxygen levels, sodium levels, and pH must be kept within normal limits. The pH of the fluid inside a healthy cell is between 7.35 and 7.45, which is slightly alkaline. *Maintaining normal pH in your cells and tissues is one of the most important things you can do for your health.* Maintaining normal pH is not optional—it is necessary. You must do it! Fortunately, this is something you can control. When your pH is normal, you will age less quickly and have more energy. When pH is not normal, cells malfunction. This means you are sick—even if you don't think you are sick. As your pH declines, your health is declining. Too many people suffer from the delusion that they are healthy, when actually they are already sick and getting sicker. When they finally arrive at a diagnosable disease, such as cancer, they are usually surprised and don't realize how long it took them to get there. The more abnormal your pH, the sicker you are, and today's cancer epidemic is just one result of abnormally low pH.

Tragically, our physicians have little understanding of the true causes of disease and have no training in how to measure health when it is in its initial decline—*but now you do*. Physicians will almost always blame your problems on getting older or on faulty genes, and not even think about the real problem of your declining pH, which has nothing to do with age or genes.

How Do Our Bodies Become Acidic?

Normal cell metabolism produces acids. A healthy diet, rich in alkalizing minerals, can neutralize these acids. However, *abnormal* cell metabolism is another matter; it produces enormous amounts of acid, and this is the major reason why so many of us are too acidic. Normal cells produce energy through a process called oxygen respiration, where fuel (mostly fats and some glucose) react with oxygen. However, our modern lifestyles impair the ability of our cells to produce energy through the normal oxidation process. Poor diets, deficient in essential energy-production nutrients such as B vitamins and magnesium, combined with our exposure to toxins such as lead and mercury, along with our lack of exercise, all work against normal energy production. When this happens, cells switch to a less complex way of producing energy called fermentation. Fermentation is a less efficient way to produce energy, and it produces lots of free radicals and lactic acid. The free radicals must be neutralized with antioxidants, but our lack of antioxidants results in systemic inflammation. The acid must be neutralized by alkaline minerals, but our modern diets are deficient in alkalizing minerals, due to mineral depletion of our soils and consumption of processed foods, so our bodies become too acidic.

The shift from normal oxygen respiration to fermentation is associated with numerous diseases, and is a major factor in accelerating the aging process. Further, once a cell loses 60 percent of its oxygen respiration capacity, this is the prime cause of cancer. (See my book *Never Fear Cancer Again*.)

Making matters worse, we consume too many acid-forming foods such as sugar, highly acidic cola drinks, excess salt, grains, dairy, and meat. On average, Americans eat far too much animal protein. When animal proteins break down in the body, they metabolize into strong acids. The bottom line is the majority of the foods most of us eat today have an acidic effect on the body. As a result, most of us suffer from chronic low-grade acidosis, which leads to chronic inflammation. Chronic inflammation drives the aging process and is the foundation of every chronic disease. This is one reason why more than three out of four Americans have a diagnosable chronic disease. Chronic stress creates acidity, and we lead stressful lives. Allergic reactions create acidity, and most of us have allergies and food sensitivities, whether we know it or not. Chronic dehydration, chronic infections, most prescription drugs, and many environmental toxins all promote acidity.

Even a small amount of acidity can lead to fatigue and feeling generally subpar. Pain is a symptom of acidity. Acidity can even make you fat. Acidic cells have a lower metabolic rate, preventing fat from being burned. To stay healthy, the body must neutralize excess acids, and healthy bodies have alkaline reserves that can be used for this purpose. However, when fermentation and our acid-forming diets deplete those reserves, the body resorts to leeching calcium and magnesium from the bones, resulting in osteoporosis. Acidosis also increases the production of free radicals, which damage DNA, cause disease, and accelerate the aging process.

Low pH and Enzymes

Abnormal cellular pH also impairs the function of enzymes, which are crucial to good health. Enzymes are little molecular machines that put molecules together or take them apart. Critical chemical reactions in the body are completely dependent on enzymes. Digesting food requires enzymes to take molecules apart, and making complex molecules, like hormones or neurotransmitters, requires enzymes to put them together. However, enzymes are pH sensitive; they generally function in a narrow pH environment. Change the pH and you change enzyme function, potentially shutting down critical metabolic machinery. For example, the liver's ability to detoxify and to produce hormones is dependent on pH-sensitive enzymes. When pH is abnormal, liver detoxification will be compromised, and this will overload the kidneys with toxins. Hormones may become unbalanced. Immunity will be depressed. Food may not be properly digested. Chemicals critical to brain function may not be produced. The pH in a cell gives chemical signals to genes, instructing them to perform or not perform certain actions. Abnormal pH will give abnormal instructions to your genes, causing cells to malfunction and make you sick.

Low pH and Cellular Oxygen

A slightly alkaline solution can absorb more than 100 times as much oxygen as a slightly acidic solution. This is why when cellular pH drops, oxygen leaves cells, and this causes a host of problems. Acidic body fluids will not support the oxygen-rich environment that the body needs for good health, and this results in chronic pain, impaired metabolism, infections, and cancer. When the fluid inside and outside the cells becomes too acidic, cell walls begin to lose their integrity. This not only damages the ability to transport oxygen into cells, it also allows toxins to enter cells. These toxins can damage DNA, causing mutations that further compromise a cell's ability to fight off disease while promoting uncontrolled cell growth and cancer. Less oxygen means less energy, but it also means increased infections. Viruses thrive in acidic, low-oxygen cells, making infection more likely. Viruses and bacteria that normally live in your body, without causing harm, will suddenly be activated in a low-oxygen environment, and this will make you sick. Our physicians then blame the "germs" and give us antibiotics, instead of normalizing our pH.

It's All About Energy

Beyond acidity and alkalinity, pH has another critical dimension in the realm of energy. While most of us don't think of it this way, the body is essentially an electronic device powered by batteries. *Each cell is a little battery, and because pH is actually a measure of voltage, your cellular pH reflects the strength of your batteries.* Remember this about your batteries:

When your batteries are strong, you are strong and healthy.

When your batteries are weak, you get tired and sick.

When your batteries are very weak, you get cancer.

When your batteries are dead, so are you.

To be healthy and live long, you must keep your batteries

    fully charged.

This is why medicine in the future will be focused more on the body's electronics and energy systems. Fortunately, you don't have to wait for the future; you can take care of your electronics now by paying attention to your pH.

Electricity plays an enormous role in almost every function in the body. One example is your heart. Physicians measure the electrical activity in the heart with a test called an electrocardiogram. Electricity generated by your cell batteries signals the heart to beat; weak batteries will cause problems with your heartbeat. Many heart patients have been given pacemakers to treat abnormal heart rhythms. Pacemakers use surgically implanted commercial batteries to send signals to the heart. A far better alternative is to strengthen your electrical system and use your own batteries as Mother Nature intended—surgery not required.

Like any electrical device, the body is designed to run at a certain voltage. Cells operate normally at a voltage of minus 20 to minus 25 millivolts (mV). There is a direct correspondence between the voltage and the pH of your cells. Minus 20 mV corresponds to a pH of 7.35, and minus 25 mV corresponds to a pH of 7.45. As you can see, keeping your pH in the normal, slightly alkaline range will maintain your voltage in the normal range. This keeps your electrical system strong and healthy and, therefore, keeps you strong and healthy. While cells normally operate at –20 to –25 mV, to make a new cell requires a much higher voltage: –50 mV. *So unless your cell batteries are working very well, and you are capable of producing and storing such a high voltage, you will be unable to make healthy new cells.* This fact is critical, because to prevent repair deficits, to heal your body, and to stay young and healthy, you must be able to produce healthy new cells. In fact, the body must produce millions of healthy new cells every second of every day.

If you are unable to create these new cells, the result is repair deficits, degenerative disease, and aging. Producing these cells requires not only the correct pH and voltage but also the correct raw materials and the absence of toxins that can impair the metabolic machinery required to build and operate the cells.

You might think a minus voltage would be weak and a plus voltage strong, but the opposite is true. In a battery, the minus end is electron-giving and the plus end is electron-accepting. That's why the minus sign in front of the voltage number means that the system is electron-giving. When it is high, your batteries are strong. This supports good health. However a *plus sign means the system is electron-stealing and your batteries are weak.* When your cell voltage is a plus, you will not be able to generate the electrons you need to operate your electrical system or to create healthy new cells—this is disease.

As long as your pH and voltage are low, you are sick, and you will not be able to get well—*you will remain chronically ill.* When your pH is low (acidic) and your batteries are weak, your body will generate lots of health-damaging free radicals. Free radicals steal electrons, damaging molecules and cells, making you sick, and causing you to age. Low-voltage cells are unable to generate the energy they need to do their regular jobs, including the movement of nutrients into the cell and toxins out of the cell. Cells will not be able to get the nutrients they need to create essential chemicals and will be unable to eliminate toxic wastes, resulting in deficiency and toxicity—the two causes of all disease. Chronic disease is always defined by low voltage. For example, cancer patients typically have a voltage of +30 mV, which corresponds to a cellular pH of about 6.5 and a urine pH of 5.7. Weak batteries and low pH are catastrophic to your health.

Measuring Your pH

Fortunately, pH is simple and inexpensive to measure; anyone can do it with some pH paper. If your pH is wrong, you can correct it. This puts you in charge of an extremely important determinant of health, contributing to *your* power to both prevent and cure almost any disease and to slow the aging process.

An indirect indicator of your body's pH is the pH of your first morning saliva and urine, before you have had anything to eat or drink. Saliva pH is an indirect indication of your cellular pH and voltage, while urine pH is an indicator of extracellular and lymphatic spaces. They should both be in the healthy range. Wet a small strip of the pH paper with the liquid and compare the color against the scale provided. Your test paper should be graduated from pH 5 to pH 8 with incremental readings (pH paper can be obtained at health food stores and at *www.beyondhealth.com*). The pH you measure will be about 0.8 pH units below what is actually in the body. So a urine or saliva pH of 6.5 will actually correspond to a pH of 7.3 in the body. Here's how to interpret your pH reading:

Below 6.5: Too Acidic
6.5 to 7.5: Healthy Range
Above 7.5: Too Alkaline

When Your pH Is Too Low (Too Acidic)

Most of us are in this category, suffering from chronic conditions ranging from tooth decay to diabetes and cancer. Chronic disease results from low pH; most chronically ill people have low pH. When your pH consistently measures below 6.5, you will begin to notice symptoms. Fatigue, chronic pain, and frequent infections can result. As your pH continues to drop, the oxygen levels in your body will drop; you will get sicker and sicker, eventually developing cancer. To be well, you must normalize your pH.

To control your pH, first pay attention to how your body is producing energy. If your body has shifted to producing most of its energy through fermentation, you need to restore proper oxygen metabolism in your cells. If you are fatigued, hypoglycemic, or experience shortness of breath upon exertion, you may be producing energy through fermentation. Restore oxygen metabolism through detoxification, regular exercise, and supplementing with B vitamins, folic acid, CoQ_{10}, magnesium, carnitine, and lipoic acid. For professional help in doing this, check Appendix C.

Avoid acid-forming foods such as sugar, grains, dairy, meat, and cola drinks. Then eat an alkalizing diet with lots of fresh fruits and vegetables, preferably organic, *and* take alkalizing supplements in highly bioavailable forms. Alkalizing supplements include calcium, magnesium, potassium, and zinc. Keep a diary of the foods you eat and record your first-morning pH. This will allow you to monitor how different foods affect your pH. As you begin eating more foods that are alkaline, and fewer acid-forming foods, you should see an improvement in your pH. To choose the right foods, see the acid/alkaline chart in Appendix A.

If diet and supplements are not able to control your pH, there are other factors to consider. Stress is one of them. Chronic stress creates acidity. Meditation techniques help to control this factor (more on this in Chapter 6). Allergic reactions create acidity. Most of us have allergies and food sensitivities, even if we are not aware of them. Find out what foods you are allergic to and take care to avoid them. Avoiding just wheat and dairy can have a major positive impact for many people. Not only are these foods acid-forming to begin with, they are also highly allergenic. Chronic dehydration, many environmental toxins, most prescription drugs, and chronic infections all promote acidity. Chronic sinus infections or dental infections contribute to acidity and need to be addressed.

When Your pH Is Normal

If you have normalized your pH, congratulations! You are on your way to reaching a strong, healthy old age. Keep monitoring your pH weekly to ensure stable results. First-morning pH should consistently run in the acceptable range. Occasional readings out-side the acceptable range are okay, but consistent readings are not. If your pH falls below the normal range, follow the recommenda-tions in the above section.

When Your pH Is Too High (Too Alkaline)

A consistently high pH can also be damaging to the body, although this is far less common than acidosis. Usually an abnor-mally high pH is an indication of an injury somewhere in the body. Sometimes chemotherapy patients have a high pH reading following therapy. Energy consumption and pH go up as the body is trying to heal itself. However, a prolonged, overly alkaline condi-tion will deplete the body of its resources, and a chronic illness will result. If your pH is consistently high, find out what is causing it, and then work to address the issue.

Remember, when your cells are healthy, *you* are healthy. When your pH drops, the voltage and oxygen drop—causing chronic pain, infections, fatigue, and cancer. When the pH inside your cells is wrong, nothing will be right. Your biochemistry and your electrical system will be compromised. Keeping your pH normal will maximize your energy and boost your immunity. Fortunately, you are in control of this critical factor, and you can use that control to choose health over disease.

To slow the aging process, maintaining normal pH is a must; it is one of the most important things you can do to maintain or restore your health. Normal pH helps to keep your body in good repair with a constant supply of healthy new cells. Acidic cells inhibit this process, causing you to age and eventually become feeble and disabled.

The Six Pathways to Health or Disease

So far, you've learned that modern aging is not a natural or inevitable condition but is evidence of disease. You've also learned that there is only one disease—cellular malfunction—and that there are two causes of disease: deficiency and toxicity. This simple mindset puts you in charge of your health because you can control your deficiency and toxicity. Here's how.

We become deficient and toxic, or avoid becoming deficient and toxic, through six major pathways. To visualize this, imagine two cities—Health and Disease. There are six major highways connecting these two cities. If you are traveling on all major highways toward Health, guess where you will end up? In Health. On the other hand, if you are traveling toward Disease on all the highways, you will end up in Disease. Most Americans are heading toward Disease because they don't know any better, but you don't have to be one of them. There are daily choices we all make that determine where we are on each pathway, in which direction we are heading, and how fast we are going. The choice between Health and Disease—between aging and rejuvenating yourself—is yours. Get yourself moving toward health on all six pathways and remain biologically young.

The Nutrition Pathway

To be healthy, the exquisitely complex metabolic machinery in your cells must receive the nutrients they need to function properly.

The Nutrition Pathway is about learning how to give your cells what they need on a daily basis. In most cases, this means changing what you eat. There is so much confusion regarding nutrition because most of the nutritional advice in the popular press is wrong. In the Nutrition Pathway chapters (Chapters 3 and 4), you'll learn how to make nutritional choices that will support health and discourage disease—choices that will help to slow down and reverse aging by supplying the raw materials your cells need to repair themselves.

The Toxin Pathway

Toxicity is one of the two causes of aging and disease. To get well and stay well, you must minimize your toxic load by learning how to reduce your toxic exposures, how to support your body's detoxification system, and how to rid yourself of previously stored toxins. In the Toxin Pathway chapter (Chapter 5) you will learn how toxins cause your cells to malfunction and what you need to do to prevent and reverse that process.

The Mental Pathway

What you put into your mind every day is even more important than what you put into your body. Every thought has a biological consequence. Putting thoughts into your mind every waking hour is one of the most important activities of your life.

Thoughts change your body chemistry, for better or for worse, in a matter of seconds. Each and every thought has a physical effect. In fact, it is not possible to have a thought without producing a physical effect. Thoughts affect our genes, our immune system, our hormones, and our digestive and other body systems. You can think yourself into getting old, and you can think yourself out of it. Every thought is a cause, and if you want to change the effects, you have to change the causes—you have to change your thoughts. In the Mental Pathway chapter (Chapter 6), you will learn how to use the incredible power of your mind to keep yourself biologically young.

The Physical Pathway

To be healthy, we must give our cells all the nutrients they need and keep them free of toxins that can harm them. To function optimally, they also need something else—to be moved and stretched. Movement helps deliver nutrients and remove toxic waste products from cells. Physical movement is a necessity for healthy life, and anyone can get the movement they need—almost effortlessly—if taught how.

Cells need to be protected from physical harm. This includes cancer-causing medical X-rays. The body also needs adequate sunlight in order to function properly. These and more, such as the effects of sleep and noise, are covered in the Physical Pathway chapter (Chapter 7).

The Genetic Pathway

Most of us think that genes run our lives, and it's true. But guess what? We run our genes. Premature aging results from changes in how genes function, which, in turn, change the way cells function. Genes don't cause aging or disease, but they play a vital role in the process. Our job is to prevent damage to our genes, quickly repair any damage that has been done, and give them the proper instructions so they will work for our greatest good (see Chapter 8).

The Medical Pathway

If you have an acute medical emergency, such as a heart attack or a traumatic injury, conventional medicine will offer the best care. However, if you have a chronic illness, such as cancer, diabetes, or heart disease, conventional medicine will be of little help, will most likely make you sicker, and may even kill you. So-called modern medicine has failed to put into clinical practice the enormous advances in science over the last century. As a result, most conventional treatments are unscientific and hopelessly outmoded—the modern-day equivalent of bloodletting. In the Medical Pathway chapter (Chapter 9), you will learn how to benefit from medicine and how to avoid being harmed by it.

The Bottom Line

✓ Accelerated aging is a disease. To slow the aging process, we need to understand what disease is, what causes it, and how to prevent or reverse it.

✓ Thinking of specific disorders as different diseases obscures the true nature of disease. There is really only one disease: malfunctioning cells. Any localized health problem is a sign of cellular malfunction throughout your body. No matter what symptoms you have, if you restore cells to normal function, you will be cured and your symptoms will go away.

✓ There are only two causes of cellular malfunction: deficiency and toxicity. Our cells will maintain and repair themselves as long as they get all the nutrients they need and are protected from toxins.

✓ We become deficient and toxic along six major pathways between health and disease. The Nutrition, Toxin, Mental, Physical, Genetic and Medical pathways will be described fully in subsequent chapters.

✓ One of the most important things you can do for your health is to maintain a normal pH in your cells.

✓ Test your morning saliva and urine with pH paper. A healthy reading is between 6.5 and 7.5. Consistent readings below 6.5 indicate you are too acidic. Consistent readings above 7.5 indicate you are too alkaline.

✓ Most Americans are too acidic. To raise your pH, restore oxygen metabolism through detoxification, regular exercise, and supplementing with B vitamins, folic acid, CoQ_{10}, magnesium, carnitine, and lipoic acid. Eliminate sugar, cola drinks, dairy products, excess salt, grains, and meat—all of which are acidic. Increase consumption of fruits and vegetables, which are alkalizing. Chronic stress, allergic reactions, chronic dehydration, many environmental toxins, most prescription drugs, and chronic infections all contribute to acidity.

CHAPTER 3

The Nutrition Pathway: The Food Challenge

*Every year over 97 percent of your body
is completely replaced, even the structure of the
DNA in your genes, reconstructed entirely
from the nutrients we eat. The quality of those
nutrients determines the quality of your
renewed cellular structure, the level at
which it can function and its
resistance to disease.*

—Dr. Michael Colgan,
author of *The New Nutrition*

> *Food is the breakthrough drug of*
> *the twenty-first century.*
>
> —Jean Carper,
> author of *Food: Your Miracle Medicine*

WHAT DOES NUTRITION HAVE TO DO WITH AGING? The answer is: everything! Americans are overfed and undernourished. Failure to supply an adequate amount of nutrients, such as vitamins, minerals, enzymes, essential fatty acids, and amino acids for optimal cell, tissue, and system function is compromising our ability to keep our bodies in good repair and working order. Most of us know that radiation damages DNA, causing cancer and aging. Few people are aware that nutrient deficiencies also cause DNA damage. In fact, inadequate nutrition is the biggest cause of accumulated DNA mutations in our cells. Deficiency of certain essential nutrients, such as vitamins B_3, B_6, B_{12}, folate, and niacin, and the minerals iron and zinc, will mimic radiation damage because they are essential to making DNA repairs. DNA damage from poor nutrition helps to explain why those who eat the fewest fruits and vegetables have double the cancer rate of those who eat the most.

The degenerative disease and accelerated aging we are experiencing today are the result of repair deficits. What do you need for making repairs? Raw materials. These raw materials are the nutrients that are in the food you eat. Yet most of us eat too much of the wrong foods, and we don't get the nutrients we need to adequately support our repair processes. *That's why the single most important thing you can do to improve your health and stay biologically young is to improve your diet by consuming more fresh, nutrient-rich, plant-based foods.*

Sadly, 20 percent of the U.S. population does not eat *any* fresh fruits or vegetables. More than 70 percent of us eat less than five servings of fresh fruits and vegetables a day, even though experts say we need at least ten servings. It's no secret that the majority of the U.S. population is consuming a diet lacking in essential nutrients. Most adult women don't meet the Recommended Daily Intake (RDI) for B vitamins, vitamin E, calcium, magnesium, and zinc. Likewise, most adult men don't meet the RDI for zinc and magnesium. Half of all Americans older than sixty are deficient in vitamins A, C, and E, even by the artificially low RDI standards. The truth is nearly all Americans are chronically deficient in at least several essential nutrients. This is catastrophic to our health, because a chronic deficiency of even one essential nutrient will cause disease and accelerate aging.

Eat for Your Cells

Although you may think of your body as a fairly stable and unchanging structure, it is not. The body is constantly discarding old cells and replacing them with new ones. This is how you stay biologically young. Your stomach lining is replaced every three to four days. Red blood cells live up to four months. The surface layer of the skin turns over every two weeks. An adult human liver replaces itself in about a year. The entire human skeleton is thought to be replaced every ten years. When worn-out cells are replaced with healthy new ones, the body stays young and can even get younger, but to become younger, every new cell must be better than the one it's replacing. All of the above requires energy, and if your cells are not producing adequate amounts of energy, repairs will not be made and you will age. Yet, due to our poor diets, most of us are chronically deficient in nutrients—such as B vitamins and magnesium—that are essential to energy production.

Let's go back to the car analogy for a moment. Say you are taking your car in for service and repairs. If your mechanic works from the right manual, uses the correct tools, and installs new original-manufacturer parts, all is like new. But if he uses second-hand replacement parts, your car will "age." *Now recall that DNA serves as the instruction manual for your cells.* When DNA is damaged, the instructions for cell repair and regeneration are compromised. Without proper instructions, new cells will be created with "birth defects" and then spread the damage throughout the tissue.

The fastest way to prevent premature aging is to improve your diet. Yet, *the single largest impediment to improving diet is that most people think they are already eating a good diet.* Because of this mass delusion, most of us need to fundamentally change our view of food and nutrition. Nothing less will get you the results you need to reverse premature aging. Most of your beliefs about diet probably come from unreliable, nonscientific sources, such as advertising, family traditions, and misinformation from the food industry—which is designed to increase its profits, not to benefit your body. Even the government's guidelines on nutrition are based more on politics than science. It's time to change that. If you already agree with most of what you see on these pages, pay special attention to the new things you are learning. Your biggest opportunity to create health and delay aging is likely to be found in these areas.

Remember, if you are not in optimal health, your body is nutrient deficient and toxic. It simply doesn't have the means to fight off aging and disease. However, as soon as you make the necessary changes, your cells will begin correcting deficiencies and toxicities and catching up on repairs. As you catch up on repairs, you will be reversing the aging process and becoming biologically younger.

What Is Food?

If you take only one piece of advice from this book, let it be this one: *eat real food*. That may sound simple, but it is not. Whether you choose to be a vegetarian or an omnivore, whether you prefer a Mediterranean or Japanese diet, to arrive at a healthy old age, *you must eat what will keep your body in proper biochemical balance*. Unfortunately, in our age of genetically altered, overprocessed, and chemically preserved make-believe foods, this is not as straight-forward as it should be. But have no fear, I will make it clear in this chapter what is and what isn't fit for human consumption. Then it's up to you to make those choices. Giving up some of your favorite treats could be daunting at first. But remember: *nothing tastes as good as being healthy feels*. As you accustom yourself to eating the right foods, your taste will adjust and your cravings for the wrong foods will diminish. Does giving up processed foods seem like a radical step to you? Perhaps it is. But did you really expect to radically improve your odds against premature aging and disease without making substantial changes?

What is the right food for a human being? Our digestive and metabolic machinery evolved in response to our prehistoric diet. This diet contained fresh fruit, vegetables, nuts, seeds, fish, and wild game. According to DNA analysis, humans have changed very little in the past 40,000 years, while our diet has changed dramatically. Our genes are still those of our hunter-gatherer ancestors, and we require the same nutrition as they did. Most of us are not getting that nutrition, but when we do get it, our bodies do very well. There are pockets of people around the world who are still eating traditional diets. These people eat few animal products and lots of fresh, whole, plant-based foods. Typically, 90 percent or more of their diet consists of plant-based foods. Chronic diseases such as Alzheimer's, arthritis, cancer, diabetes, heart disease, osteoporosis, and other common afflictions of modern societies are virtually nonexistent among these populations. John Robbins, in his book *Healthy at 100*, described some of these people, noting the complete absence of processed foods in their diets.

Avoiding processed foods is important for several reasons. First, processing causes the loss of critical nutrients and the formation of toxins. Second, processed foods rob the body of electrons and weaken your cell batteries. Fresh, whole foods are electron donors, helping to keep your batteries charged. Processed foods have lost most of their voltage. To metabolize them, the body must supply voltage from its own batteries.

Medical researchers estimate that our ancestors consumed four times more nutrients than we do today, and for some nutrients, such as trace minerals, that number is twenty or even fifty times higher. At the same time, the changes in our environment and lifestyle make our need for nutrients the highest ever. We have created an oxidizing environment that increases our need for antioxidants, and our enormous exposure to environmental toxins requires extra energy and materials for the body's detoxification processes. *Compared to our ancestors, our need for nutrients is sharply up while our intake of nutrients is sharply down.* The resulting deficiencies are causing an epidemic of chronic disease and accelerated aging.

Most people are unaware of the unprecedented burden that our exposure to environmental toxins is placing on our bodies, dramatically increasing our need for nutrients. Meanwhile, the concept of eating for nutrition and health is not the norm in our society. Most people make food choices based on what tastes good, or what is convenient, and they consume staggering quantities of biologically inappropriate sugar, grains, dairy, and processed foods. Yet, the data clearly show that countries that consume more fresh vegetables and fewer processed foods have longer life spans and less disease.

How Our Poor Food Choices Began

Our food problems started with the Industrial Revolution in the late 1700s. Coal-fueled steam engines introduced machine-based manufacturing and changed life forever, as people moved off the farms and into the cities to work in factories. To feed all those people in big cities, food had to be processed so it could be stored for long periods and transported to distant markets. Thus began a period of drastic changes in our diet that are still ongoing. Most of our calories today come from "foods" that did not even exist only a few hundred years ago. Processed foods like white flour, refined sugar, and white rice were considered "perfect" solutions. Their shelf life is almost forever. They supply calories, produce energy, and take away your hunger—but they lack essential nutrients. Soon, other methods of processing to extend shelf life were developed, such as canning, freezing, adding preservatives, and later irradiating.

Processing is the ultimate robber of nutrition. You get shelf life and convenience but you lose nutrition, in some cases almost all of it. Not only are nutrients lost, but toxins are generated as well as added, creating both deficiency and toxicity—the two causes of disease and accelerated aging. Toxins are added to processed foods in the form of preservatives to give shelf life, artificial colors to make food look more appealing, artificial flavors to replace lost flavor, flavor enhancers to increase flavor, salt to mask bad flavors and improve color, chemicals to help retain moisture, and processing aids to make the manufacturing process go more smoothly. Ninety cents out of every food dollar is spent on these toxic, nutritionally poor, disease-causing processed foods. Some people eat little else, and it is destroying their health and accelerating their aging.

Personally, I find it depressing to go to a supermarket (I call it the disease store) and watch people pay good money to load up their grocery carts with every imaginable disease. Often, there will be no real food whatsoever in the cart. It will be filled with bread, cookies, baked goods, and breakfast cereals; canned goods; frozen pizzas; milk, cheese, and dairy products; fruit drinks and sodas; fruits and vegetables sprayed with toxic chemicals; produce too old to retain much nutrition; refined sugar in many forms; processed oils; hydrogenated fats; processed meats; artificial colors, flavors, and preservatives; farmed fish and feedlot-raised meat. The cart will be loaded with cancer, diabetes, heart disease, arthritis, Alzheimer's, osteoporosis, and accelerated aging. Then, after decades of spending a lot of money to buy aging and disease, somehow it is still a surprise when we finally get what we paid for.

The Big Four—What Not to Eat

The American diet can best be described as bizarre. No one in history has ever consumed such a diet. Modern diets are so bad that Dr. Carl Pfeiffer, a medical pioneer and author of the breakthrough book *Mental and Elemental Nutrients,* concluded that, "The average human diet, nutritionally unfit for rats, must be equally unsatisfactory or even more so in meeting human needs." The foods most of us eat will not support healthy life in rats, yet we feed them to our children. This is why our children are old and sick, and why they are projected to be the first generation in more than two hundred years to die at a younger age than their parents.

To eat a better diet, first understand that the Standard American Diet (SAD) will not sustain healthy life. Nor will the strictest adherence to any diet help you if you are misinformed about which foods are really healthy. Our bodies need a major change from the way most of us eat, plus supplementation with high-quality vitamins, minerals, and other nutrients. To start, eliminate the Big Four from your diet. What I call the Big Four are "foods" you definitely should not eat. They are: *sugar, wheat, processed oils,* and *dairy/ excess animal protein.* These foods are primary causes of accelerated aging and every known chronic disease.

Sugar Is More Dangerous Than Alcohol and Tobacco

It is hard to think of a single food that is more dangerous and more destructive to human health than sugar. Sugar not only makes you sick with everything from the common cold to cancer, *sugar makes you old.*

Sugar elevates insulin, and high insulin sets off a cascade of disturbances at the cellular level that accelerate the aging process. Even a modest increase in blood sugar generates a flood of free radicals, causing inflammation and damage to genes and tissues. Sugar disrupts the metabolism of hormones, fats, carbohydrates, proteins, vitamins, and minerals. This suppresses immunity, digestion, nerve function, cell repair, and hormone and enzyme production, throwing the body into biochemical chaos and accelerating the aging process. In addition, *metabolizing sugar is acid-forming in the body, lowering your pH and damaging your cell batteries.* This is why Nobel laureate Linus Pauling called sugar "the most hazardous foodstuff in the American diet." To avoid being old and sick, stop eating sugar.

Refined sugar is so harmful to human health it should be outlawed like street drugs, or at least made a controlled substance like alcohol and tobacco. Sugar acts like a drug and is addictive, similar to alcohol, heroine, and cocaine. Most Americans have a sugar addiction, but only a few realize it. The more sugar you eat, the more sugar you will want. Some people try to wean themselves off sugar gradually. This is generally not a good way to do it, since eating even a little sugar makes you crave more. Children should not be allowed to purchase or consume products containing sugar.

A 2012 study published in *Nature* looked at the toxicity of sugar and concluded that the sugars found in processed foods and drinks are to blame for our increasing rates of chronic disease, accelerated aging, and premature death. The researchers recommended that the government regulate the use of sugar. They urged the Food and Drug Administration to remove sugar from the list of foods "generally regarded as safe."

Even one teaspoon of sugar will damage your health, and most Americans eat and drink more than 450 calories, or roughly twenty-two teaspoons, of added sugar every day—triple what they consumed three decades ago. Few people are aware of the various ways sugar sneaks into their diets, hiding in breads, sauces, and other processed foods. Many "healthy" choices—bottled juices, breakfast cereals, and granola bars—come loaded with sugar. Oftentimes, it appears in disguise on food labels under names like sucrose, glucose, fructose, maltose, hydrolyzed starch, invert sugar, corn syrup, and honey.

Like alcohol and tobacco, sugar is an addictive, toxic substance that is responsible for a whole range of chronic diseases that are reaching epidemic levels around the world. According to the study in *Nature*, sugar changes metabolism, raises blood pressure, critically alters the signaling of hormones, and causes significant damage to the liver. At the same time, sugar makes people crave sweets even more. The problem with sugar is not just the "empty calories" that make you fat. Sugar is in fact very toxic to the body. Whether or not you gain weight from eating sugar, the health effects are devastating—and you age.

Sugar AGEs You Faster Than You Can Say, "Advanced Glycation End Products"

Yet another way sugar ages us is through the formation of dangerous compounds called *advanced glycation end* products (AGEs). It has been known for decades that diabetics age faster than nondiabetics, suffering problems in the eyes, brain, vascular system, and kidneys. The reason for this is the high sugar levels in the blood of diabetics and a process called *glycation*. Glycation happens when a sugar chemically bonds to proteins or certain fats to form AGEs. However, you don't have to be a diabetic to be damaged by glycation. Eating even a teaspoon of sugar is sufficient to raise the sugar content of your blood and create a lot of AGEs.

AGEs form inside the body whenever you increase the sugar content of the blood. The sugar then reacts with proteins, fats, enzymes, and even the DNA in your cells. A breakfast of eggs and orange juice puts both sugar and protein into the blood at the same time, forming AGEs. Any protein meal followed by a sugary dessert will create AGEs.

Glycation fundamentally changes functional proteins so they can no longer accomplish their mission in the body, and the damage is permanent. Glycation causes body tissues to lose their natural flexibility, stiffening joints, hardening arteries, weakening heart muscles, and causing skin to wrinkle and to lose its elasticity. *Glycation ages you, and it happens every time you eat the deadly metabolic poison called sugar.*

AGEs are absorbed into various body tissues, where they remain for long periods, causing oxidative damage. This initiates chronic inflammation. The result is massive, systemic inflammation throughout the body, and inflammation is the foundation of every chronic disease. Making matters worse, oxidative stress and inflammation facilitate the formation of even more AGEs. This further increases your risk of Alzheimer's, diabetes, heart disease, stroke, kidney failure, neurological deterioration, cataracts, retinal damage, and vision loss.

Immune cells try to get rid of AGEs. However, if you eat a lot of sugar and create a lot of AGEs, the immune system becomes overworked and less able to protect you from infections and cancer. Glycation damages enzymes. Disabled enzymes shut down critical functions inside cells. AGEs are produced internally, but you can eat them as well. AGEs form in foods during the cooking process, particularly as foods brown. Every time you eat foods that have been caramelized or meats that have been browned, you increase the amount of AGEs in your body. Foods likely to supply AGEs include bacon, hot dogs, cured and smoked meats, and baked beans. Even toast will contain AGEs.

Note that any food that spikes your blood sugar will cause glycation. This includes natural sweeteners like honey, maple syrup, agave nectar, brown rice syrup, and fruit juices. Fresh whole fruit is okay in moderation. The sugar in whole fruit is less concentrated than sugar in fruit juice, and we only metabolize about 30 percent of it because we do not chew our food thoroughly enough. This makes the whole fruit safer than the juice.

It is now well established that glycation plays an important role in the aging process, as well as in diseases including cancer, diabetes, heart disease, kidney disease, and Alzheimer's. If you must cook food, cook at lower temperatures as in steaming, poaching, stewing, and slow cooking. Avoid high-temperature cooking, as in barbecuing, broiling, frying, grilling, and roasting. Do not brown or blacken foods. Most of all, if you don't want to make yourself old and sick, avoid sugar.

As If You Needed Another Reason to Stay Away from Sugar—Fructose

Fructose is a type of sugar present in fruits, honey, agave nectar, maple syrup, corn syrup, high fructose corn syrup, and crystalline fructose. *Although all sugars contribute to aging, the latest research shows fructose to be especially damaging to health.*

Unfortunately, fructose is very common in our modern diets. Almost every kind of processed food contains fructose, and typical supermarket sweets carry monster doses. All of the fructose you eat is broken down in the liver, compared to only 20 percent of glucose (another common sugar). That's a lot of work for your liver! What's more, fructose metabolism produces a number of toxic waste products. One of these, uric acid, raises blood pressure and can damage your kidneys. Fructose converts to fat much faster than other dietary sugars, and it contributes to VLDL ("bad" cholesterol). The excess fat causes insulin resistance and nonalcoholic fatty liver disease. Insulin resistance progresses to metabolic syndrome and Type 2 diabetes. Then, as if all the fat you gain from eating fructose wasn't enough, fructose interferes with leptin, the hormone that suppresses appetite, and this causes you to overeat.

The American diet of processed foods is loaded with fructose, and the result is our ever-increasing rates of obesity, diabetes, heart disease, nonalcoholic fatty liver disease, and accelerated aging. If you want to stay biologically young, maintain a healthy weight, and radically reduce your risk of diabetes, heart disease, liver disease, and cancer, then you must eliminate all refined sugars from your diet and keep your daily consumption of fructose to a minimum, from all sources, including fresh fruit and honey.

It is best to stay away from sweeteners, natural or otherwise. As you incorporate more fresh whole foods into your diet, your sweet cravings will diminish, and your natural energy will rise. When you must use a sweetener, stevia is your best choice. Use raw honey in moderation and avoid all syrups including agave nectar, which is almost all fructose. In fact, most agave nectar contains more fructose than high fructose corn syrup.

A Special Look at High-Fructose Corn Syrup

High-fructose corn syrup (HFCS) is in most of the processed foods manufactured in the United States, including breads, breakfast cereals, lunchmeats, yogurts, soups, sodas, condiments, and desserts. It's the cheapest form of sugar on the market, and as long as it is legal, there is no reason for the processed food manufacturers not to use it. However, there are excellent reasons for you not to eat it if you care about your health. On top of being a refined sugar, HFCS, which is made from genetically modified, chemically processed corn, comes with its own unique set of poisons. One of the many chemicals used to turn corn into cornstarch and then into HFCS, glutaraldehyde, can burn holes in the human stomach, even in small doses. Yet, small amounts of glutaraldehyde remain as a residue in the HFCS, and over time, this toxin can accumulate in your body.

Chemical processing also leaves HFCS with residual mercury. A 2009 study in *Environmental Health* found that between one-third and one-half of all HFCS-containing products on the market tested positive for mercury contamination. How much mercury? Enough to consume five times the recommended maximum daily dose simply by eating the average amount of HFCS in the American diet. Mercury causes Alzheimer's, cancer, high blood pressure, depression, arthritis, and many other diseases. Today, many people test high for mercury, and most have no idea how to protect themselves. This is a big source of mercury that isn't even on most people's radar. A simple solution is to *stop* eating HFCS. Since most processed foods contain HFCS, avoid processed foods, and always remember to read labels carefully.

Don't Touch That Cola

If you drink any kind of soda or sweetened drinks, the best and easiest thing you can do to stay young is to switch to pure water once and for all. A 2012 study in the *Journal of General Internal Medicine* found that one can of diet soda a day increases the risk of heart disease by 43 percent. The same study showed similar liver damage between soda drinkers and alcoholics. There is no doubt that soft drinks—both sugar-sweetened and sugar-free—are disastrous to our health. How? Here's a short list.

Obesity. Studies have concluded that every can of soda you drink per day increases your risk of being overweight. Children are at special risk. Consuming lots of fructose will cause more cells to turn into belly fat when the child's fat cells mature.

Diabetes. A 2004 study in the *Journal of the American Medical Association* concluded that women who drink one sugary soda a day double their risk of developing Type 2 diabetes compared to women who drink less than one a month.

pH. The sugar and phosphoric acid found in most sodas have an acidic effect on the body, lowering cellular pH and voltage.

Pancreatic cancer. A 2010 study in *Cancer Epidemiology, Biomarkers & Prevention* determined that drinking two or more soft drinks a week almost doubles the risk of developing pancreatic cancer compared to drinking none.

Premature aging. An increasing number of studies are showing that the phosphoric acid added to colas for its tangy taste causes premature aging. Our phosphorus balance influences the aging process, and drinking sodas upsets this balance. The result is accelerated aging, shriveling of the skin and muscles, and damage to the heart and kidneys.

Osteoporosis. The acidic effect of sodas drains calcium from the bones, putting you at risk for osteoporosis. Several studies have found a strong association between bone fractures and the amount of cola drinks consumed.

Dental problems. Not only do soft drinks cause cavities due to the high sugar content, they also erode tooth enamel. Phosphoric acid—present in most sodas—causes tooth enamel erosion, even with minimal exposure. Dentists are reporting teen patients whose front teeth are completely eroded by the acids in sodas.

Fertility. Men who drink a quart or more of sodas a day lower their sperm counts by 30 percent. Women who drink just one diet cola a day increase their risk of miscarriage by 38 percent, and four or more colas a day increases the risk by up to 78 percent.

Toxicity. Artificial sweeteners are toxic, poisoning the brain, kidneys, digestive system, and liver.

Wheat: A Ten-Thousand-Year-Old Mistake

Most people are aware that white flour is nutrient-deficient and unhealthy. To make white flour, the whole grain is stripped of more than twenty essential nutrients, including 72 percent of its zinc and 85 percent of its vitamin B_6. When a handful of these nutrients are added back, the flour is called "enriched." White flour is mostly starch and quickly metabolizes into sugar, causing all the same problems as sugar. Like sugar, white flour causes an increase in blood sugar and insulin, and produces a flood of pro-inflammatory chemicals and free radicals. All of these accelerate aging. The average American consumes about 200 pounds of this deadly junk food every year.

When I ask people if they eat white flour, many claim they don't. When I point out that white flour is a major ingredient in many of their favorite foods, they are shocked to discover how much of it they do eat. Some people don't realize they are consuming white flour when they are eating breakfast cereal, bread, a dinner roll, a bagel, a pretzel, a cookie, a pancake, pasta, pizza, or a piece of pie. It's all white flour, and it's all inflammatory and enormously damaging to human health, disrupting vitamin and mineral metabolism and hormone balance. Even products labeled as "whole wheat" or "whole grain" often contain mostly white flour.

While the problems with white flour are well known, most people are unaware that grains themselves are a problem, and that *wheat is the worst grain of all.* The wheat we eat today differs from what our ancestors ate. Even the baked goods made by our great-grandmothers back in the 1940s were fundamentally different from those made today. Modern wheat has been hybridized to achieve a higher yield per acre and a higher protein content. Few thought this high-protein wheat would present a problem, and hybridized wheat was introduced into commerce without testing for safety. As it turns out, that wasn't such a good idea. Small changes in the structure of a protein molecule can spell the difference between a healthy nutrient and a toxin, and proteins in modern hybridized wheat are having a toxic effect. High-protein wheat supplies higher amounts of two classes of proteins—gluten and lectins, which both present special challenges for human metabolism.

Gluten, found in barley, rye, and all types of wheat, is highly inflammatory. It causes diarrhea and abdominal pain, as well as brain inflammation, which can result in depression, poor cognitive function, and dementia. Even if you are not allergic to gluten, getting it out of your life will reduce the inflammation in your body. Meanwhile, researchers have estimated that as much as half the population may now be metabolically reactive ("allergic") to gluten. Gluten reactivity manifests as a wide range of health problems including chronic depression, chronic fatigue, common colds, eczema, fibromyalgia, irritable bowel syndrome, lupus, thyroid disease, and rheumatoid arthritis. Meanwhile, most people suffering from gluten sensitivity are completely unaware of the root cause of their symptoms. Immune reactions to gluten produce free radicals and inflammation. They also make the body more acidic. Gluten sensitivity is causing an epidemic of premature aging and chronic disease. Choosing a diet that does not promote inflammation is absolutely essential for a long, disease-free life; eliminating gluten is a near foolproof way of getting a powerful inflammation promoter out of your life.

Grains, as well as other foods, also contain proteins called lectins. Research presented in the *FASEB Journal* (2008), *Gut* (2000), *Lancet* (1999), *Pediatric Allergy and Immunology* (1995), *British Journal of Nutrition* (1993), and numerous other sources indicate that lectins may be the biggest problem with grain consumption. Lectins are powerful natural insecticides that plants use to protect themselves. Lectins attach to receptor sites on the cell membranes of bacteria and fungi and disrupt their function. This protects wheat and other grains from insects and infection, but humans have exactly the same receptor sites. Hybridized, high-protein wheat is especially high in lectins, and this is having a devastating effect on human health.

When we eat wheat, the lectins damage our gastrointestinal tract, creating holes in the gut tissue that make it more permeable to larger molecules. This is called leaky gut. Once the gut is leaky, undigested molecules, including gluten, enter into the bloodstream. The immune system sees these molecules as invaders and attacks them, creating inflammation and allergies. Increased intestinal permeability is now recognized as causing a wide variety of chronic inflammatory and autoimmune syndromes, including inflammatory bowel diseases, celiac diseases, multiple sclerosis, and eczema. In fact, lectins can do direct damage to the majority of tissues in the human body, and this helps to explain why chronic inflammatory diseases are more common in wheat-consuming populations. Even in small quantities, lectins have profoundly adverse effects on the entire body. At exceedingly small concentrations, lectins stimulate the production of pro-inflammatory chemicals such as interleukins 1, 6, and 8 in intestinal and immune cells. The inflammation created by lectins damages DNA and accelerates aging.

Lectins damage the thymus gland, which is essential to immunity, and directly damage immune cells in the blood. They also damage the thyroid gland. Lectins have the ability to pass through the blood-brain barrier and directly damage brain cells; they can also attach to and damage the myelin sheath coating on nerves. Lectins also exhibit insulin-like properties, which can cause insulin resistance (diabetes) and weight gain. They signal genes, causing production of chemical compounds such as epidermal growth factor, which, when elevated, increases the risk of cancer. Lectins stimulate platelet stickiness and blood clots, contributing to the risk of heart attack and stroke.

Unfortunately, lectins are highly stable molecules. They are resistant to degradation through a wide range of pH and temperatures. They survive cooking, sprouting, fermentation, and digestion. We are now consuming a lot of high-lectin wheat, and it is accumulating in our tissues, putting a continuous toxic load on us. Ironically, whole wheat contains more lectins than white flour, and, in this regard, *may be an even bigger threat to our health.*

Grains were a very minor part of the human diet until about 10,000 years ago. In the last 130 years, grain consumption has sharply increased, along with our rates of chronic disease. Now grains represent about half of all the food consumed. All plants contain natural toxins to protect them from viruses, bacteria, fungi, and predators. Our genes are well adapted to handle the toxins in fruits and vegetables, but not so for the relatively recent addition of the special toxins in grains. Anthropological evidence indicates that when we started eating grains, our health declined: infant mortality increased, life span shortened, infectious diseases increased, and bone disorders and dental decay appeared. Another reason for this is that, aside from lectins, grains contain phytic acid, which prevents the absorption of calcium, copper, iron, magnesium, and zinc, causing mineral deficiencies. Eating grains also causes insulin to spike, which creates a cascade of harmful reactions in the body. The process of metabolizing most grains, especially refined grains, is acid-forming. *This lowers cellular pH, damages your cell batteries, leaches minerals from your bones and teeth, and accelerates aging.* Quinoa, whole oats, buckwheat, and Japonica rice are better choices because they are mildly alkaline-forming.

Grains do contain some useful nutrients, but cooking is usually necessary to make grains edible. This creates both deficiency and toxicity problems. Cooking significantly diminishes nutritional value, while yeast-containing baked goods are toxic. Many studies have linked bread and other bakery products with cancer. This is due to the carcinogenic mycotoxins they contain. Mycotoxins are metabolic waste products of the yeast used to make bread.

Most people think of wheat as a good food. However, there is sufficient evidence that it is instead a toxin and a major cause of aging and disease. Anyone with a chronic illness should avoid all products containing wheat. In the interests of living a long, disease-free life, most people would do well to eliminate or at least minimize the consumption of grains—most especially wheat.

Change Your Oil

When it comes to your health, *virtually any oil you buy at the supermarket is the wrong oil.* This includes all hydrogenated oils, canola, corn, cottonseed, peanut, safflower, soybean, sunflower, and even most olive oils. *If you want to be healthy or recover from a chronic disease, you need an oil change.*

Cell membranes (the walls enclosing the interior of the cells) are constructed with oils. These membranes perform many critical tasks, including the exacting job of correctly regulating what goes in and out of a cell—controlling the delivery of essential nutrients like oxygen and the removal of metabolic wastes. These complex tasks can only be performed well if the membranes are constructed of the correct oils. *The processed oils we buy in our supermarkets are the wrong oils!*

To keep ourselves in good repair, we build millions of new cells every second of every day. Unless the proper oils, in the correct ratios, are available when a new cell is being created, the body will use whatever is available from your diet or from your old cells. Think of building a new house out of cardboard instead of high-quality plywood because the plywood is unavailable, but the cardboard is. Almost all the processed food we eat, such as salad dressings, baked goods, chips, breakfast cereals, fast foods, and restaurant foods are made with biologically incorrect oils. Because the wrong oils interfere with transporting nutrients into cells and toxic wastes out, they create deficiency and toxicity in your cells, resulting in cellular malfunction and disease.

The wrong oils also compromise the electrical properties of cells. Properly constructed cell membranes act as electrical capacitors, storing electrical energy for the cell. Recall that cells that normally operate at −20 to −25 mV need to build up and store the much higher −50 mV voltage in order to construct a healthy new cell. *Faulty cell membranes diminish the strength of your cell batteries to the point where it is not possible to construct the healthy new cells that are necessary to keep your body in good repair. This is why processed oils make you old.*

Properly constructed cell membranes are made out of very specific oils called essential fatty acids (EFAs). There are two categories of EFAs: omega-3 and omega-6. Both are healthy, and both oils must be available when new cells are constructed, but it is important that these oils be consumed in the proper ratio to each other. Humans evolved on a diet that had a near equal 1:1 ratio of omega-6 and omega-3 oils. However, due to the proliferation of supermarket oils, most Americans consume far too much omega-6 and too little omega-3s. The current ratio in our diet is about 20:1, and for some people it's as bad as 50:1. About 90 percent of the U.S. population is deficient in omega-3 fatty acids. A 1991 study in the *World Review of Nutrition and Dietetics* showed that 20 percent of us have so little omega-3 in our blood that it cannot be measured by standard tests. Biologically speaking, this is a disaster!

The imbalance of omega-6 and omega-3 oils in our diet will both initiate and perpetuate inflammation. This is highly significant because inflammation is a common denominator of all chronic disease. Both classes of EFAs produce body chemicals called prostaglandins. Inflammatory prostaglandins are produced from omega-6 fatty acids; they suppress the immune system and increase inflammation, heart disease, cancer, and aging. Excess omega-6s dramatically lower the amount of vitamin E in the body, which increases free-radical damage to DNA and tissues, promoting the growth and metastasis of tumors. In addition, fatty acid imbalance causes the clumping of red blood cells, which slows down blood flow, restricts blood flow to the smaller capillaries, and results in poor oxygen delivery to cells.

When sufficient omega-3 oils are present, anti-inflammatory prostaglandins are produced, and these offset those from the omega-6s. Anti-inflammatory prostaglandins from omega-3s suppress inflammation, tumor development, blood pressure, water retention, blood platelet stickiness, and cholesterol levels.

While the primary reason for this enormous imbalance of 6s and 3s is the excessive consumption of supermarket oils, a secondary reason is the decrease in the consumption of "real" fish, meat, and eggs. For example, most of the salmon and many of the other fish available today have been farmed in artificial environments. Farmed fish are grain-fed, as opposed to the normal diet they would consume in their native oceans and rivers. As a result, they contain the wrong fatty acid ratios because grains are high in omega-6s. The same holds true for beef and chicken, which are fed grains that change their fatty acid ratios.

Consider that a real egg, from a hen eating a natural diet, contains about 300 milligrams of the omega-3 fatty acid DHA (docosahexaenoic acid). Standard, grain-fed, supermarket eggs average only 18 mg of DHA, while being high in omega-6s. These omega-3-deficient, industrially produced foods are damaging our health.

Nearly all cattle are shipped to feedlots prior to slaughter to "fatten up." If you eat this grain-fed beef, as most Americans do, you worsen your omega-3-to-omega-6 fatty acid ratio. Natural beef is rich in omega-3s, but grain-fed beef is rich in omega-6s. If you choose to eat beef, eat grass-fed, organic beef, which is available online and at health food stores. Just eating organic meats is not good enough. That just means the animals were fed organic grains. The meat contains fewer pesticides but still has the wrong fatty acid ratio; grass-fed is what you want.

To increase the amount of omega-3s in your diet, include flaxseed oil and flaxseeds. Flaxseeds, freshly ground in a small coffee grinder, make an excellent addition to fresh salads. Healthy omega-6 to omega-3 ratios are found in rich sources of EFAs like green leafy vegetables, nuts, and seeds.

Not only do supermarket fats and oils supply too much omega-6 and too little omega-3, they are also highly processed. Commercial processing subjects them to heat, chemicals, and oxidation, significantly changing their molecular structure and making them toxic to the body. Most supermarket oils undergo a bleaching and deodorizing process to make them crystal clear and to extend shelf life. This usually takes place at high temperatures, at which massive transfat formation occurs and powerful toxins called lipid peroxides are formed. There is no safe level of lipid peroxides or transfats. Processed oils precipitate a chain of oxidative events in the body that can severely damage cells. Another problem is that about 40 percent of edible oils, especially soy and corn oils, contain solvent residues from their manufacture, contributing to our toxic overload.

Yet another problem occurs when processed oils are burned by cells as fuel to create energy. To burn the fuel, enzymes must combine it with oxygen. But enzymes are designed to fit and interact with very specific molecules, and the misshaped oil molecules from overprocessed supermarket oils will not fit the appropriate enzyme. You won't get the energy you need because you are supplying the wrong fuel!

Because processing deprives oils of their natural antioxidants, toxic preservatives are added to processed oils. The fats we call hydrogenated oils are especially dangerous, and they are found in everything from baked goods to breakfast cereals to peanut butter. They are man-made fats containing a variety of unnatural molecules, including transfats, all of which are toxic to your body and interfere with energy production. Some products are now being labeled as "transfat free," but this can be deceptive. Transfats only have to be disclosed on the label if the food contains more than 0.5 grams per serving. Even that amount is too much and toxic, but to avoid listing transfats, or to claim "transfat free" on their label, food manufacturers simply adjust the serving size until the transfat content falls under 0.5 grams per serving. Thus, modern food labels often have serving sizes that are much smaller than the amount you would normally consume. So be sure to read food labels carefully.

Never eat anything containing any hydrogenated oils, which are sometimes listed as "margarine" or "vegetable shortening."

A 2011 study published in *Neurology* confirmed that people with diets high in omega-3 fatty acids are less likely to have the brain shrinkage associated with Alzheimer's disease than people whose diets are low in omega-3s. Those with diets high in omega-3 fatty acids and in vitamins C, D, E, and B also had higher scores on thinking tests than people with diets low in these nutrients. The study also showed that people with diets high in transfats were more likely to have brain shrinkage and lower scores on the thinking and memory tests than people with diets low in transfats.

To get adequate oxygen and essential nutrients into your cells and to be able to store the voltage required to build new cells, cell membranes must be constructed with the proper oils. Avoid supermarket oils, all hydrogenated oils, and all food products containing these oils. Avoid grain-fed animals, eggs, and fish—they are too rich in omega-6s. Instead, fill your grocery cart with fresh organic vegetables, fruits, raw nuts, wild-caught fish, and organic grass-fed meats. Anti-aging oils include olive, coconut, palm, flaxseed, and fish oils, but these must be high-quality oils, and most brands do not measure up. (See Appendix C for good sources.) Use high-quality olive oil for cooking and for salad dressings (most olive oil is adulterated with toxic oils). Flaxseed oil is also excellent for salads. Use both olive and flaxseed oil for good health. Without the correct oils in your diet, you will get sick and accelerate aging. If you want to prevent or reverse premature aging, you need an oil change!

Skip All Dairy and Watch Out for Excess Animal Protein

Americans have been terribly misled into consuming milk and dairy products, and far too much animal protein. We are among the world's highest consumers of milk products, and we also consume about ten times too much animal protein. Protein is an essential nutrient, required to construct hormones, enzymes, and other indispensable molecules, as well as structural tissue. Without protein, life cannot be sustained. However, animal protein, in excess of the amount needed for growth, promotes aging and disease. Unlike plant protein, the animal protein in milk and meat metabolizes to strong acids. *This lowers the pH of your cells, robs your teeth and bones of minerals, and makes your cell batteries weaker.*

The Recommended Daily Intake (RDI) for *total* protein is 50 to 60 grams per day. Many Americans get twice this amount. Our average consumption of animal protein alone is about 70 grams per day. *Americans average more animal protein than the RDI for total protein.* By contrast, most rural Chinese, who are far healthier than we are, average 7 grams of animal protein per day (about the amount contained in one egg). Averaging 7 grams or less per day of animal protein is a worthy goal—approximately one egg or a piece of fish or meat the size of the palm of your hand. The remainder of the RDI should be plant protein from vegetables, nuts, seeds, sprouts, legumes, and avocados.

Got Toxic Milk?

Consuming milk is both unnatural and unhealthy. If this is the first time you are hearing this, it may be shocking, but nowhere in nature does one species drink the milk of another or drink milk after weaning. Only humans do these things, and we pay a heavy price in the form of heart disease, osteoporosis, diabetes, infections, arthritis, allergies, cancer, and accelerated aging.

Most Americans grow up believing that milk, cheese, yogurt, and even ice cream are vital parts of a healthy diet. The first time someone suggested that dairy products were not healthy, I thought that person was crazy. Unfortunately, we've all been misled into believing we need milk for calcium and strong bones. The truth is that milk damages bones. Milk and dairy products do very little to sustain health. Even back when most of us were farmers, traditional milk from one's own cow was not a healthy food choice, but then it wasn't a deadly poison either. Modern milk, on the other hand, is a highly toxic, processed, and allergenic make-believe food. No one should be drinking milk or consuming products made with milk.

Modern industrial milk is a toxic soup. It is loaded with more than fifty biologically active hormones; more than fifty powerful antibiotics; dozens of allergens, pesticides, herbicides, PCBs, and dioxins (up to 200 times the safe levels); and blood, pus, feces, solvents, viruses, excessive bacteria, and even radioactive compounds. Yummy!

Of the dozens of biologically active hormones contained in your milk, one is the powerful growth hormone IGF-1 (insulin-like growth factor 1). IGF-1 instructs cells to grow. Instructing cells to grow may be fine for the infant, for whom the milk is intended, but in adults, it promotes cancer. IGF-1 is especially known to be a factor in the rapid growth and proliferation of breast, colon, and prostate cancers. Cows treated with synthetic growth hormones such as rBGH produce milk that is especially high in IGF-1. Drinking only one glass doubles the amount of IGF-1 in your body, and the biological effects are significant. Most of the milk used to make ice cream comes from rBGH-treated cows, and one serving of ice cream gives you twelve times as much of this powerful cancer accelerator as you would get in one serving of milk, because the IGF-1 gets concentrated in the cream. IGF-1 is like rocket fuel for cancer.

In addition to hormones, most ice cream is also loaded with sugar and other toxic chemicals, including artificial colors, flavors, and processing aids. Most ice cream also contains carrageenan, which is used as a thickening, emulsifying, and stabilizing agent. Carrageenan has an inflammatory and immunosuppressive effect on the body, and degraded carrageenan is a carcinogen. Because of this, most manufacturers will use undegraded carrageenan, but there is evidence it degrades in the digestive system. Carrageenan is also used in yogurt, custards, jellies, cream cheese, cottage cheese, and other dairy products, as well as chocolate products, pie fillings, salad dressings, soups, and soymilk; as a fat substitute in processed meats; and in toothpaste.

Almost all milk is pasteurized and homogenized. This processing substantially changes the chemical and physical properties of the milk, and, for many reasons, makes it less nutritious, more toxic, and more carcinogenic. We are all paying a very high price for the misguided advice put out by the dairy industry.

Pasteurized milk is an acidic food. Most Americans are eating too many acidic foods already, and milk throws their systems further out of balance. In *Fit for Life: A New Beginning,* author and nutritionist Harvey Diamond states, "It is a well-established fact that the high protein content of meat and dairy products turns the blood acidic, which draws calcium out of the bones. This causes the body to lose or excrete more calcium than it takes in. The deficit must be made up from the body's calcium reserve, which is primarily the bones."

Think about this: milk causes calcium losses and osteoporosis. Yet people with osteoporosis are told to consume more milk! Calcium is indeed needed, but drinking milk causes you to lose calcium. Vitamin D is critical for calcium metabolism, which is why most milk is "fortified" with vitamin D. However, a study in a 2001 *American Journal of Clinical Nutrition* article found that those who consumed the most milk actually have the lowest vitamin D levels. Industrial milk is not a good source of bioavailable calcium, and the vitamin D used to fortify it is the wrong form of vitamin D.

Some people think that raw organic milk is a safe choice, but here's another problem: milk protein itself. The largest and most comprehensive nutrition study done to date is "The China Study," conducted by world-renowned nutrition researcher Dr. Colin

Campbell, who wrote a book with the same title. Campbell found that *the most powerful cancer driver of all was milk protein.* Casein, the predominant protein in cow's milk, promotes cancer at every stage in the cancer process.

Casein in cow's milk is also difficult for humans to digest. Because undigested casein molecules are highly allergenic, an estimated half of our population is allergic to milk. Dairy allergies present a serious health problem, leading to numerous disorders. Continual immune reactions to dairy protein will put the body in a state of chronic inflammation.

As if all that isn't bad enough, cow's milk contains viruses that promote cancer, especially leukemia and lymphoma. More than half the dairy herds in America are infected with these viruses, and people living in areas near the infected herds suffer significantly more leukemia.

When I tell people not to drink milk, they often ask, "Where will I get my calcium?" Seventy percent of the world's people do not drink milk. Where do they get their calcium? They get it from plant foods, as do gorillas, elephants, horses, and even cows, which have bigger bones than we do. Green vegetables, such as kale, broccoli, and collard greens, are loaded with bioavailable calcium.

Paul Nison, in his book *The Raw Life,* stated, "Dairy is the cause of most disease in the world today." When Dr. Russell Bunai, a prominent Washington, DC, pediatrician, was asked in an interview what single change to the American diet could provide the greatest health benefits, he replied, "The elimination of milk products."

Have Your Steak on the Side

Excess animal protein accelerates aging and promotes chronic, degenerative, and autoimmune diseases. A high animal-protein diet changes the ratio of estrogens in the body, shifting the balance to those that stimulate cancer. People who are on high protein diets to lose weight need to be aware of this danger. Animal protein is also rich in a fat called arachidonic acid, and studies have linked arachidonic acid to tumor growth and metastasis.

Meat, especially red meat, contains iron. While iron is an essential nutrient and is needed for oxygen transport in the blood, excess iron is toxic. The way to measure your iron levels is with a blood test for ferritin. Any doctor can order this test. If your ferritin is high, you have a problem and need to reduce your iron level.

Animal protein can be safely and beneficially consumed in small quantities. However, the source is important. Processed meat is especially problematic. A 2010 study in *Circulation* concluded that one extra serving of processed meat (hot dogs, bacon, or hamburgers) per day increased the risk of dying from heart disease by 21 percent and the risk of dying from cancer by 16 percent. A similar quantity of unprocessed meat raised the heart disease risk by 18 percent and the cancer risk by 10 percent. If you choose to eat meat, make sure it's unprocessed and organic. The fish you eat should not be farmed, and your eggs should be organic as well. A good rule is to use animal protein as a condiment, not as a main course. There is no need to consume animal protein at every meal or even every day. Most of your protein should come from plant-based foods. Most people have been so conditioned to think of meat and dairy as their source of protein, they don't even think about the protein in plant foods. Consider this: calorie-for-calorie, spinach has 20 percent more protein than beef.

Excess animal protein invites chronic disease. Dr. Campbell's research linked the intake of animal protein with obesity, Alzheimer's, osteoporosis, diabetes, heart disease, and kidney and eye disorders, among other ailments. Plant protein does not have a cancer-promoting effect, and large amounts can be safely consumed. Here are some ways to cut down on animal protein:

Introduce more primarily vegetarian meals.

Build meals around fresh raw salads as the main course. You can add a small amount of high-quality animal protein or protein-rich sprouts to your main-course salad.

Avocados are a good source of vegetable protein, contain healthy fats, and can be used to replace meat in meals.

Nuts and seeds (raw and soaked/sprouted) are a good source of protein and healthy fat, which can be satisfying.

Lentils can be easily adapted to replace ground beef in Mexican recipes, shepherd's pies, meatballs, and stuffed peppers.

If you do eat meat, make sure it is not grilled, charred, or browned in any way. When fat drips into an open flame, dangerous carcinogens called polycyclic aromatic hydrocarbons are formed. All proteins cooked at high temperatures have been proven to cause cancer in laboratory animals. Barbecuing is the worst way to prepare meat because of both the open flame and higher temperatures. When you cook meat, it is best to cook it at a low temperature, such as in a crockpot.

To slow and reverse the aging process, reduce the animal protein in your diet. At least 90 percent of your protein should be derived from plant foods such as vegetables, whole grains, lentils and other legumes, seeds, nuts, and sprouts. Fish and seafood were tradition- ally healthy forms of animal protein, as they closely resemble the diet of primitive man. However, they are now loaded with toxins, because we have poisoned the oceans. Fish at the high end of the food chain, such as Chilean sea bass, tilefish, swordfish, and tuna, are generally the most contaminated and should be avoided. A 2004 study in the *Annals of Internal Medicine* linked these fish to autoimmune disorders, cancer, endocrine system disorders, heart disease, and neurological disorders. An occasional small portion of fresh fish may be okay to consume, but farmed or canned fish are not options. Farmed fish contain too many toxins and the wrong fatty acid ratios. Canning destroys nutrition and adds toxins. Best advice: Severely limit how much fish and seafood you eat. Especially avoid the most heavily contaminated species.

A Common Food Additive That Makes You Old: Salt

Beyond the Big Four, there are other health-damaging substances in our diet, and salt is one of them. Common table salt is a big prob- lem, but for a different reason than most people think. Salt is sodium chloride, and when you eat too much salt, it results in an excess of sodium and a relative deficiency of potassium. This upsets the ratio of sodium to potassium inside our cells, causing cellular malfunction, disease, and accelerated aging. *Too much salt makes you old.*

According to the Centers for Disease Control and Prevention (CDC), 90 percent of Americans consume too much salt, and up to 90 percent of our salt comes from processed foods. Average salt consumption in America is 3,400 mg per day, and some of us consume more than 10,000 mg per day. Consider these numbers in light of a 2010 study in the *New England Journal of Medicine*, which estimated that cutting salt intake by 3,000 mg per day would prevent enough heart attacks and strokes to save $24 billion from the national health care tab. Excess sodium in the diet is a disaster for our electrical system. Salt has an acidic effect on the body, lowers pH, and forces more sodium into cells. This weakens our cell batteries, damages the body's electrical system, and, among other problems, causes heart palpitations.

We need sodium to help our nerves function properly, to aid nutrient absorption, and for maintaining the right balance of water and minerals in our bodies. The human body requires about 220 mg of sodium per day. *One teaspoon* of refined salt contains 2,300 mg of sodium—about ten times what we need. Try to keep sodium intake to less than 1,000 mg per day or less than a half teaspoon. (In special circumstances, such as excessive sweating or chronic diarrhea, higher levels may be necessary.) Even the government is concerned about excess sodium consumption and is now recommending that most adults in the United States eat no more than two-thirds of a teaspoon of salt each day; only about 5 percent of us are actually doing that.

Natural foods, which are rich in potassium and low in sodium, are what we were designed to eat. Unfortunately, we have changed to a sodium-rich diet of processed foods, and it is making us sick. Even eating at a "healthy" salad-bar restaurant can be a health hazard. Consider this: If you have a bowl of split-pea soup, you will consume 1,430 mg of sodium. A serving of a typical "healthy" nonfat Italian salad dressing adds another 1,350 mg. Two "healthy" low-fat muffins add another 1,400 mg. A serving of mushroom marinara sauce on your hot pasta adds another 318 mg. Choosing a couple of the salad offerings adds another 400 mg, and chocolate pudding for dessert adds another 177 mg. This adds up to a whopping 5,075 mg of sodium—at just one meal—and the body needs only 220 mg per day.

Some of the biggest sources of sodium are products made from grains, such as bread, pasta, and pizza crust. Tomato sauce and cheese add even more sodium. One slice of whole-wheat bread typically contains about 100 mg. There are 200 mg in one cup of cornflakes, and 709 mg in two ounces of turkey-breast lunchmeat. Still more can be found in processed vegetables, including vegetable-based soups and sauces and canned vegetables, not to mention potato products such as chips and fries. There are 390 mg of sodium in a half-cup serving of canned peas and 780 mg in one cup of canned vegetable beef soup. One cup of low-fat milk contains 107 mg of sodium, and one ounce of cheddar cheese contains 180 mg. Many people don't think of these foods as containing much sodium at all.

When your sodium intake is too high, your bones get weak. For every 2,000 mg of sodium you eat, you will lose about 25 mg of calcium in your urine. Unless you replace the lost calcium—and most people don't eat enough bioavailable calcium to do that—then eating an average of 5,000 mg of sodium per day could result in calcium losses as high as 2.5 percent of your skeleton annually. At that rate, you will lose 25 percent of your bone structure in only ten years. Since bone loss is progressive, older people tend to have weak bones, and today even young people suffer from weak bones. Osteoporosis is just one more "disease of aging" that we ourselves create and can easily prevent.

Excess sodium also increases the risk of high blood pressure, which is a major cause of heart disease and stroke. In fact, people who consume more than 4,000 mg per day double their risk of stroke compared to those consuming less than 1,500 mg. Other ramifications of excess sodium include chronic fatigue, neurological disorders, cancer, weight gain, impaired immune function, and premature aging. Research reported in a 2013 *Nature* concluded that excess salt triggers an abnormal immune response, which is capable of causing autoimmune diseases such as multiple sclerosis, psoriasis, and rheumatoid arthritis.

Mother Nature tells us the balance of sodium and potassium we need. Human milk contains three times as much potassium as sodium. Yet we are consuming four times as much sodium as potassium. Fast foods are loaded with salt. It takes a lot of awareness to eat a low-salt diet, but you can do it. In restaurants, soups often contain a lot of salt: avoid them. Many restaurants use too much salt: request less. Read labels carefully. To increase potassium, eat more fresh fruits, vegetables, nuts, and seeds. Foods that are high in potassium include bananas, oranges, avocados, tomatoes, broccoli, lima beans, melons, cucumber, papayas, mangos, kiwi, and spinach. These same foods contain many other nutrients that our bodies need to stay healthy and biologically young.

Other Food Additives That Make You Old: Glutamates

Glutamates are a class of compounds known as excitotoxins that are used in processed foods, fast foods, and in restaurants to enhance the flavor of the food. The best-known glutamate is monosodium glutamate (MSG), but there are others. Glutamates produce enormous amounts of free radicals in the body, and free-radical damage causes aging. Regular consumption of glutamate-containing foods will age you.

Most of us are exposed to glutamates daily because they are in about 80 percent of all processed foods and many restaurant foods. Glutamates are cleverly disguised on food labels with words such as "natural flavors, spices, hydrolyzed vegetable protein, vegetable protein, sodium caseinate, textured protein, soy protein extract," and others. This is why a restaurant menu that says "No MSG" may still be serving you food loaded with glutamates. Even baby formula can contain glutamate in the form of caseinate. When you start to look for it, you may be shocked at how often you will find glutamates. They are everywhere. Commercial pizza and most fast foods are known to have a lot. Glutamates damage the brain and nervous system. They are also known to cause diabetes, obesity, and heart attacks.

GMO Foods: An Impending Disaster

There is a reason genetically modified (GMO) foods have been outlawed in countries around the world: They are dangerous! GMO foods are a threat to human health and to all life on the planet. Yet Americans are consuming them by the ton. Genetic engineering happens in a lab where genetic material from one species is inserted into that of another species, in a way that couldn't happen in nature. This process can and does result in many unintended consequences. For example, it can change the nutritional content of the food, making it far less nutritious. It can make the food more allergenic. Unique toxins have been created in these plants that no one would even think to look for, and that's just the tip of the iceberg. Each generation of GMO crops interacts with other organisms in the environment. This creates more opportunities for unwanted side effects that could ultimately affect every living thing on the planet with catastrophic consequences. This damage may take years to manifest and is difficult to trace back to the GMO food.

Animal studies from around the world have shown GMO crops to be dangerous, causing damage to the liver, heart, lungs, kidneys, adrenal glands, intestines, spleen, and pancreas. They also shorten life and promote massive tumors. The introduction of foreign genes changes the entire nature of plant biology, turning food into a disguised poison that can potentially contaminate the genetic code of other plants and animals, including us. Genetically modified plants can be designed to produce internal pesticides that we then eat. Such is the case with Monsanto's GMO corn. The corn's DNA has been altered by inserting a gene from *Bacillus thuringiensis,* a soil bacteria called Bt, which produces the pesticide Bt-toxin. Monsanto claimed the toxin is harmless to humans because it's destroyed during digestion. It isn't. A 2011 Canadian study in *Reproductive Toxicology* found Bt-toxin in the blood of hundreds of women, including pregnant women and their babies.

Glyphosate, the active ingredient in Monsanto's herbicide Roundup, is the most common weed-killer in the United States. It is heavily used on GMO crops. Glyphosate has been linked to miscarriage, infertility, and premature aging in animals raised on GMO feed. A big problem is that glyphosate gets into the root system and contaminates a plant from the inside. You can't wash it off. Further, it stays in the soil for years, killing beneficial microbes and promoting disease-causing pathogens. When you eat one of these GMO plants, the glyphosate ends up in your gut, where it destroys beneficial bacteria. Your immune system and your health are totally dependent on the beneficial bacteria in your gut, so this can wreak havoc with your health. Glyphosate also reacts with critical micronutrients in the soil, making them unavailable to the plant. This substantially reduces the nutritional quality of the plant. For example, nutrients such as iron, manganese, and zinc can be reduced by as much as 80 to 90 percent in GMO plants, and they are already low to begin with because of soil depletion.

A 2012 study in *Food and Chemical Toxicology* was the first long-term study on the health impacts of GMO corn, and the results were truly alarming. The researchers fed Monsanto's Bt corn to lab rats. The rats developed serious liver and kidney damage, and exhibited increased and earlier development of tumors. The animals also showed allergic and inflammatory responses, potentially linking GMO crops to a wide range of disorders, from arthritis and inflammatory bowel disease to multiple sclerosis. They also had elevated T cells, which you typically see in people with a variety of diseases, including allergies. Genetic engineering is mad science, and it's absolutely unnecessary. There are safe, organic farming methods that allow us to grow sufficient food without poisoning our environment and our bodies.

Here is a list of the genetically modified food crops that are commercially produced in the United States today: corn, soybeans, canola, cotton, sugar beets, and papayas grown in Hawaii. GMOs are used extensively in foods like popcorn, canola oil, cottonseed oil, soy sauce, frozen pizza, frozen dinners, dry cereal, baby formula, canned soups, cookies, and ice cream.

Since in the United States the FDA doesn't require GMO foods to be labeled or tested for safety, *the simplest way to avoid them is to buy whole, certified organic foods.* By law, foods that are certified organic must never intentionally use GMO organisms and must be produced without artificial pesticides and fertilizers. Certified organic animals must be reared without the routine use of antibiotics, growth promoters, or other drugs. Unfortunately, even organic crops are now being contaminated with GMOs, which is why even organic soy and corn are not necessarily safe to eat.

The Bottom Line

✓ The most important thing you can do to improve your health and stay biologically young is to eat a good diet. Most people believe they are already eating a good diet, but unfortunately they are mistaken. Many foods assumed to be healthy are not. Not if you want to avoid disease and premature aging.

✓ A good diet is composed primarily of unprocessed, non-GMO, fresh, nutrient-rich plant foods.

✓ The most damaging foods you can eat are The Big Four: sugar, wheat, processed oils, and dairy/excessive animal protein.

✓ Refined sugar is a deadly poison. It ages us and makes us sick by setting off a cascade of metabolic disturbances. Sugar is so dangerous and destructive to human health, it should be outlawed or at least made a controlled substance. High fructose corn syrup (HFCS), found in many processed foods, is even more destructive than regular sugar.

✓ Glycation ages the body and plays a role in many chronic diseases. Glycation is a chemical process in which high levels of sugar in the blood damage body proteins so that tissues lose their flexibility. This results in stiff joints, hardening of the arteries, weakened heart muscle, and wrinkles. Glycation is also caused by cooking food at high temperatures so that they get browned or even charred. Avoid barbecuing, broiling, frying, and grilling; it's healthier to steam, poach, stew, or slow cook.

✓ Human health has declined since grains became a substantial part
of our diet about 10,000 years ago. Most people would do well
to eliminate or at least minimize consumption of grains. Avoiding
wheat has become a must. Modern wheat has been hybridized
to contain dangerously high levels of gluten and lectins. Yeast-
containing bread and other baked goods are especially harmful
due to the carcinogenic mycotoxins they contain.

✓ Processed oils found in supermarkets are toxic and should be
avoided. This includes canola oil and even most olive oil. Most
of us are in need of an "oil change." The American diet is too
high in omega-6 fats and too low in omega-3 fats. This leads to
inflammation and a host of related diseases. To change your oil,
eliminate supermarket oils, grain-fed animals, conventional eggs,
and farmed fish (high in omega-6s), and include flaxseed oil and
flaxseed as well as green, leafy vegetables, some nuts and seeds,
eggs from chickens allowed to forage in open pastures, and
grass-fed meats. Transfats should be avoided, yet many labels
saying "transfat-free" are deceptive. If the label lists hydrogenated
fat, margarine, or vegetable shortening, the product contains
transfats. Anti-aging oils include olive, coconut, palm, flaxseed,
and fish oils as long as they are correctly and carefully produced
and handled.

✓ Consuming the milk of another species is unnatural and
unhealthy. Casein, the predominant protein in cow milk, promotes
cancer. It is also difficult for humans to digest, which has led to
dairy allergies in up to half the population. Dairy is linked with

heart disease, diabetes, infections, arthritis, allergies, cancer, osteoporosis, and accelerated aging. Modern milk is a toxic soup, not a food. Get your calcium from green vegetables.

✓ Animal protein can be safely and beneficially eaten in small quantities, but most Americans consume far too much. Of the 50-to-60 recommended grams of daily protein, only about 10 percent should come from animals; the rest should come from plant foods: vegetables, seeds, nuts, sprouts, legumes, and avocados. Excess animal protein unfavorably alters hormone ratios, is pro-inflammatory, and has been linked with many chronic diseases. Red meat often causes excess iron, which is toxic. Avoid farmed fish and canned fish. Fish should be eaten only occasionally, if at all, as they have become too polluted.

✓ Our bodies were designed for a high potassium/low sodium diet, but our modern diet is low in potassium and high in sodium. This unfavorable ratio weakens our cell batteries and damages the body's electrical system. Excess sodium also causes calcium to be lost in the urine, increasing the risk of osteoporosis. Excess salt is linked to chronic fatigue, neurological disorders, cancer, weight gain, impaired immunity, and aging. Keep salt intake to less than half a teaspoon a day. We get most of our salt, about 90 percent, from processed foods. Restaurant foods and fast foods are usually high in salt.

✓ Monosodium Glutamate (MSG) is the one of many sources of glutamates found in about 80 percent of processed foods, and in fast foods and restaurant foods. Glutamates enhance flavor, but they are excitotoxins that produce a flood of free radicals in the body (free radical damage causes aging) and are especially harmful to the brain and nervous system. They also cause diabetes, heart attacks, and obesity. On food labels, glutamates are disguised with words like natural flavors, spices, hydrolyzed vegetable protein, vegetable protein, sodium caseinate, textured protein, soy protein extract, and others.

✓ Genetic modification is science gone mad. Genetic material from one species is inserted into that of another in a way that can't happen in nature. This has all kinds of unforeseen consequences which threaten everything from nutrient content of food to the future of the planet. The genetically modified crops produced in the U.S. today are: corn, soybeans, canola, cotton, sugar beets, and papayas grown in Hawaii. The simplest way to avoid GMO foods is to buy whole, certified organic foods. However, organic soy and corn are not necessarily safe to eat as they are easily contaminated by GMOs.

CHAPTER 4

The Nutrition Pathway: The Right Foods

The key to health is to make sure the cells have the raw materials they need to maintain a healthy chemical balance. . . . If the cells are healthy, consequently the whole body is in good health.

—Gary L. Samuelson, author of *The Science of Healing Revealed*

Whereas animals in the wild with DNA closest to ours consume almost 100 percent raw plants, the humans of the Western world today are consuming virtually none.

—J. Morris Hicks, author of *Healthy Eating, Healthy World*

C UTTING BAD FOODS OUT OF YOUR LIFE is one step in the right direction; putting good foods in is another. A diet consisting primarily of fresh plant food is an anti-aging diet. *Sadly, only one out of ten Americans is meeting the current USDA guidelines for consumption of fruits and vegetables.* Federal guidelines recommend nine servings of fruits and vegetables per day. Even this is too little, and nutrition experts recommend more. Gorillas are amongst our closest relatives in the animal kingdom, with DNA similar to ours, and they consume almost 100 percent raw plants. Most of us consume less than 10 percent of our calories from raw plants, and many less than 5 percent. This is a big mistake!

The key to health is to make sure your cells are getting everything they need to do their jobs. Recall from a previous chapter that to keep yourself in good repair and biologically young, cells have a grocery list of essential nutrients that must be supplied regularly. Every day you create hundreds of billions of new cells. Constructing them properly requires a bewildering array of complex chemicals, which must come from your diet. Modern processed-food diets fail to supply these needs. The result is our epidemic of chronic disease and accelerated aging. By contrast, raw plant food can supply a balance of proteins, carbohydrates, and oils, as well as the vitamins, minerals, phytochemicals, and fiber that we need, which is why eating unprocessed foods is essential.

To prevent aging, raw, fresh vegetables, along with fruits, nuts, seeds, sprouts, and legumes, must be the foundation of your diet. Hundreds of studies show that eating more fresh fruits and vegetables reduces the risk of all types of disease. Very simply, plant foods contain nutrients and phytochemicals that protect your cells and keep them in good repair. To get the nutrition you need, at least 80 percent of your diet should be raw; remember that cooking food destroys critical nutrients and creates dangerous toxins.

Eating more fruits and vegetables actually decreases your appetite for fatty, processed foods. The best vegetables to keep the body biologically young are the cruciferous vegetables: broccoli, cabbage, brussels sprouts, mustard greens, kale, and cauliflower. Other good vegetables include carrots, onions, beets, and spinach. Good fruits include avocados, cherries, blackberries, blueberries, raspberries, pineapples, watermelon, kiwis, mangos, plums, and honeydew melons. Fruits are healthy, but they should be consumed in moderation because of their high sugar content. Fruit juices should be avoided because they rapidly increase blood sugar and insulin.

The critical anti-aging nutrients in vegetables can be made even more bioavailable by juicing or "blenderizing." Use a juicer or powerful blender to mechanically break the tough cell walls of the plants to release more nutrition. This way you can get three times the nutrition from the same food than if you chewed it. Chewing makes only a fraction of the nutrition available, and most people don't chew well. A combination of juicing and blenderizing is best. Juicing is less filling because it removes the fiber, which allows you to consume more vegetables and get more nutrients. Blenderizing retains the fiber, and most of us don't get enough fiber. There are many suitable juicers and blenders on the market. Experiment with a variety of vegetables and drink a glass of vegetable juice every day. It's best to drink your juices immediately after they are prepared. A healthy combination includes carrots, celery, tomatoes, kale, spinach, broccoli, and beets. An apple or a slice of lemon adds flavor.

Cooking for Your Cells

How you prepare your food is critical. Cooking food is another major change we have made in our diets since Paleolithic times, and it is a major obstacle to meeting our bodies' nutritional needs. Cooking reduces the availability of many of the precious nutrients and phytochemicals. Cooking carrots, for example, can destroy 75 percent of vitamin C, 70 percent of B_1, 50 percent of B_2, and 60 percent of B_3. Produce such as apples, beets, cabbage, and cauliflower lose most of their anticancer activity when they are cooked. The higher the heat and the longer the cooking time, the more nutrients are lost. If necessary, the best way to cook vegetables—for example, broccoli or spinach—is to lightly steam or quickly stir-fry them.

Raw Is Best

As much as possible, eat raw foods. Cooking deactivates health-sustaining enzymes in the food. Although the human body makes its own enzymes if they are not available in the food, manufacturing these extra enzymes puts stress on the body, depleting essential nutrients and contributing to aging and disease. Unfortunately, we are eating fewer raw foods than ever before. According to USDA statistics, over the last century, average consumption of fresh apples declined by more than three-fourths, fresh cabbage by more than two-thirds, and fresh fruit by more than one-third. During that same period, consumption of processed vegetables went up hundreds of percent, and consumption of processed fruits went up by 1,000 percent.

If you must eat cooked foods, eat something raw first, such as a salad, before the main course. Cooked food appears to be so alien to the human system that it provokes an immune response, as if you were being exposed to a virus. Scientist Udo Erasmus, author of *Fats and Oils,* wrote, "When cooked food is eaten, a defense reaction occurs in the tissues of the stomach and digestive tract. This reaction is similar to the reaction we find in infections and around tumors and involves the accumulation of white blood cells, swelling, and a fever-like increase in temperature of the stomach and intestinal tissues."

This reaction does not occur if raw food is consumed prior to eating the cooked food.

Cook at a Low Temperature

If you are going to cook, how you cook makes a difference. Cooking food at high temperatures, as in grilling, frying, broiling, and barbecuing, not only destroys nutrients but poisons the food with powerful carcinogens. The high heat of grilling causes chemical reactions with the proteins in red meat, poultry, and fish, producing carcinogenic compounds called heterocyclic amines. Another class of cancer-causing agents, polycyclic aromatic hydrocarbons, forms when the juices from meats drip into the open flame or another heat source, then rise in the smoke and contaminate the meat. Barbecuing is the worst way to prepare meat because of both the open flame and higher temperatures. Meat that has been blackened is the most carcinogenic of all—*never* eat any food that has been blackened. Even well-done meat is highly contaminated. *All proteins cooked at high temperatures have been proven to cause cancer in laboratory animals, and numerous studies have shown that people who eat meat cooked at higher temperatures have higher cancer risk.* When you cook meat, it is best to slow cook it at a low temperature using a crockpot.

Retire Your Microwave

Microwave ovens are found in almost every kitchen, yet micro-waved food is a dangerous health hazard. Microwaving not only destroys most of the nutrition, it also introduces toxins that interfere with critical processes in the body. Eating microwaved food damages cell-to-cell communication, stresses the immune system, and lowers the oxygen-carrying capacity of the blood, all of which causes aging and disease. Research reported in the April/May 1995 *Nexus* by Dr. Hans Hertel and Dr. Bernard Blanc of the Swiss Federal Institute of Technology found pathological changes in the blood of volunteers who ate microwaved food. Blood samples from test subjects demonstrated impaired immunity due to decreased lymphocytes (white blood cells) and decreased hemoglobin. Decreased hemoglobin lowers the oxygen-carrying capacity of the blood, making less oxygen available to cells, causing fatigue and increasing the risk of cancer. In fact, any food that has been cooked or defrosted in a microwave oven can cause changes in the blood similar to the pathological changes we find in cancer.

Microwaving food massacres its nutrients. A 2003 study in the *Journal of the Science of Food and Agriculture* reported that broccoli lost 97 percent of its antioxidants when cooked in a microwave. By contrast, only 11 percent was lost when steamed. Foods today are already nutrient deficient, so why make them worse by cooking them in a microwave? If you must cook, steaming is generally the least damaging way to cook.

Putting It All Together:
The Anti-Aging Diet

Vegetables, including sprouts, must be the foundation of an anti-aging diet. The fiber, enzymes, phytochemicals, minerals, and many other nutrients they contain are essential. Dozens of anti-aging compounds have been identified in plants. As much as possible, have organic salads, vegetables, vegetable juices, and sprouts for breakfast, lunch, and dinner. Since all vegetables have different kinds and amounts of nutrients, it is best to eat a variety. Leafy dark-green vegetables such as kale, spinach, and Swiss chard are especially high in nutritional content. Whenever possible, buy organic fruits and vegetables. It is even more important that animal protein be organic. Eating organic makes a difference. Studies show that people who eat organic foods have virtually no pesticides in their urine, while those eating nonorganic foods often exceed safety levels.

Following is a list of vegetables to include in your anti-aging diet:

arugula	cucumbers	peas
asparagus	eggplant	peppers
beets	garlic	radishes
broccoli	green beans	scallions
brussels sprouts	kale	sea vegetables
cabbage	lettuce	spinach
carrots	mustard greens	squash
cauliflower	okra	Swiss chard
celery	onion	turnips
collards	parsley	watercress

The foods listed above are highly curative and protective. You want a diet high in fresh, organic fruits and vegetables and high in omega-3 fatty acids. Nongluten grains such as buckwheat, millet, brown rice, quinoa, and amaranth are okay in moderation, but grains are not a natural dietary choice for humans. Legumes and lentils are good sources of plant protein. Occasional small portions of high-quality animal protein, such as organic eggs, can be added. Sprouts are an excellent food choice and highly recommended on an anti-aging diet. However, store-bought sprouts are too often contaminated with dangerous bacteria and mold. Growing your own sprouts is best, and it is simple to do. Sprouting is a fast, inexpensive way to produce high-quality food in your own kitchen. Books or web sites on raw foods usually have a section on sprouting. There are also entire books written on the subject. If you are not sprouting already, I invite you to learn a few basics and get started.

While we may call the above an anti-aging diet, in reality it is the diet humans are intended to eat. Premature aging is a mistake. To prevent and reverse premature aging, as much as possible, follow these rules:

Avoid processed foods.

Be wary of restaurant foods, unless organic and raw.

Choose organic produce and meats.

Eat a primarily plant-based diet.

Get on a high-quality supplement program.

Avoid processed, supermarket fats and oils.

Consume a balance of healthy omega-6 and omega-3 oils.

Include high-quality flaxseed and olive oils in your diet.

Avoid sugar and wheat, and minimize grains.

Avoid dairy products.

Limit alcohol and coffee.

Avoid foods high in mold such as peanuts, corn, and dried fruits.

Avoid barbecued and microwaved foods.

Minimize animal protein, and it must be organic.

Juice or blenderize fresh vegetables every day.

Protect Your DNA

Protecting DNA from damage, and repairing damage as it occurs, is critical to preventing aging and disease. Accumulated DNA damage ages us and underlies most of the conditions that kill us, such as heart disease, cancer, and Alzheimer's disease. Many fruits and vegetables, such as cantaloupe, cherries, sweet potatoes, kale, carrots, and spinach, contain carotenes that protect against DNA damage. Animal experiments and human experience have shown that high amounts of dietary carotenes have a rejuvenating effect on the body, supporting healthy skin, hair, and eyesight, and protecting from disease. Olive oil helps to protect DNA from oxidative damage. Phytochemicals in tea inhibit DNA damage. Green tea has been found to reduce the incidence of disability, heart attacks, and strokes, and promote mental sharpness. Herbs such as silymarin (milk thistle seeds) and ginkgo biloba also contain powerful anti-aging compounds. Beyond Health Age Defense Formula offers extraordinary protection (for more information, see Appendix B).

Garlic Is Great for Your Arteries

It has been known for thousands of years that garlic is a healthy food. More recently, numerous studies have shown that raw garlic and garlic extract protect your arteries and guard against heart attacks and strokes. Garlic reduces cholesterol and triglycerides, lowers blood pressure, prevents platelet aggregation, and helps dissolve blood clots. Garlic is a powerful antioxidant; it neutralizes free radicals present in the blood and helps preserve the heart muscle, increasing your chances of surviving a heart attack.

A Berry for Your Thoughts

A Harvard study in the 2010 *Annals of Neurology* found that cognitive aging (the loss of the ability to think, reason, and remember) is delayed substantially in older people who eat greater amounts of berries. Flavonoids in berries have powerful antioxidant effects and also fight inflammation, which, along with stress, contributes to cognitive decline. Berries are only one source of essential nutrients that keep your brain biologically young. The more fruits and vegetables you eat, especially the colorful varieties, the sharper your mind will stay as you advance in years. Flavonoids and anthocyanidins—chemical compounds that give fruits and vegetables their pigment—help repair the brain cells damaged by oxidative stress and inflammation. Some of the most colorful and deeply colored fruits and vegetables, like black and red grapes, cranberries, blackberries, blueberries, raspberries, red cabbage, red onion, and eggplant, are the richest in anthocyanidins.

Nuts Cut Cancer Risk

Nuts are a good food choice. They can be a small part of an anti-aging diet, but many nuts, such as cashews and peanuts (which are not really nuts), may be too contaminated with mold to be safe. Eat only organic, whole, and unprocessed nuts. The best choices are almonds, macadamias, Brazil nuts, and walnuts. According to research at the U.C. Davis Cancer Center, which was presented at a 2010 annual meeting of the American Chemical Society, walnuts affect several genes that control tumor growth and metabolism, cutting cancer risk and also slowing the growth of tumors. Walnuts have also been linked to better brain function.

I recommend soaking raw nuts and seeds before you eat them or use them in recipes. Soaking removes anti-nutrients—naturally occurring chemicals that interfere with nutrient absorption—

usually in the skin of the nut. Soaking also helps remove the impurities and softens and rehydrates dry nuts and seeds, making them easier to digest. For this reason, I recommend soaking even skinless nuts, like macadamias and cashews, for anywhere from twenty minutes for softer nuts to a few hours for harder nuts, like almonds and Brazil nuts.

Water

Drinking an adequate amount of water is essential to good health. Studies show that most people are chronically dehydrated, especially those older than fifty. Even a small amount of dehydration will affect all the chemistry in your body. Water hydrates the body and helps to remove toxins. Most experts recommend drinking at least eight glasses per day. However, the water has to be pure. Tap water is not appropriate. I recommend a reverse osmosis system for drinking water. Boiling the water doesn't purify it from industrial contaminants, like lead, arsenic, and fluoride, to name a few. On the contrary, as some of the water evaporates, the chemicals in the remaining water become more concentrated.

How Food Becomes Nutrition (or Not)

It may not be enough to simply eat all the right foods. Many steps are involved in liberating the nutrients from the food you eat and transporting these nutrients to your cells where they are needed. Proper digestion requires that a progressive series of processes go well in order to turn your food into vital nourishment. Otherwise, even the healthiest food can become toxic waste.

Digestion

How you eat is critical. If you eat too fast or under stress, or if you eat the wrong combination of foods at a meal, the food may not be properly digested. *If the food isn't properly digested, you can't get the full nutritional value. Further, undigested food promotes the creation of dangerous toxins that poison the body.* The resulting deficiency and toxicity contribute to aging and disease.

Digestion begins in the mouth. Each stage in the process of digestion requires a specialized set of enzymes. Digestive enzymes farther down the gastrointestinal tract rely on the enzymes in your saliva to initially break down the food. You can think of them as workers along an assembly line. If a team of enzymes has not finished its task by the time the food moves from the mouth into the stomach, then the next team of enzymes cannot properly complete its own task, and the whole process is compromised. This is why one of the best things you can do for your health, after selecting and preparing healthy food, is to chew your food thoroughly. Most people don't.

Food Combining

Proper food combining means eating those foods together that require the same chemical environment for their digestion. Each type of food requires a different combination of digestive juices to be properly digested. For starchy foods, such as grains in any form (bread, pasta, rice, etc.) and potatoes, the body needs an alkaline environment to break down and use the nutrients they contain. For proteins, on the other hand, it requires a highly acidic environment. If you eat both a starch and a protein at the same time, expect problems. As your body pours alkaline components into the digestive system in order to break down starches, it also releases acid to digest proteins. The acids and alkalis neutralize each other so that nothing gets digested properly. Your valuable digestive enzymes are wasted as more and more are poured into the system in a strained attempt to deal with this situation. Your body is working so hard that you may feel sluggish. Starches require less time in the stomach before moving on to the intestinal tract, where much of their digestion occurs. When starches enter the stomach with proteins, which require a longer time there, they get held up. The starch begins to ferment, creating toxins and causing gas, bloating, abdominal discomfort, acid indigestion, poor nutrient absorption, and many other problems. Since most people in our society eat protein along with starch (meat and potatoes), indigestion and acid reflux have become normal. Americans spend more than $2 billion a year on antacids!

Fruits generally contain all of the enzymes necessary for their digestion, so they can and should pass through the system in much less time than either starch or protein. Some fruits, such as melons, are only in the stomach for fifteen to twenty minutes. Others are there slightly longer, but none as long as starch, let alone protein. When you eat a big meal and then have fruit for dessert, your stomach is already full and mixing in enzymes as it churns the meal. Along comes fruit, which is designed to pass right through, but now it cannot. It is stuck behind the meal. When fruit is forced to remain in the stomach with a starch, the mixture ferments and creates toxins that spread throughout the body. If the fruit remains in the stomach with a protein meal, digestion is again impaired, and the protein putrefies, similarly resulting in powerful toxins being released into your body. With impaired digestion, you cannot reap the nourishment from the food consumed, so you may be hungry again soon. You eat more to satisfy your hunger, but all you are doing is adding toxins and withholding nutrients yet again.

Our digestive systems were not designed to eat what has become the "normal" diet of protein-and-starch meals. These foods may still be enjoyed, but learning a new way to eat them will maximize the benefit you receive from them. If you eat three meals a day, have one fruit meal, one starch meal, and one protein meal (not necessarily animal protein). Fruit is a wonderful morning food (as long as you don't have a blood sugar problem). Since the stomach is empty, fruit can pass right through, and the body can easily absorb all of its life-giving vitamins, minerals, trace minerals, and enzymes to make us flourish. Eating fruit in the morning also extends the time the body has to "rest" since active digestion is not required. Lunch can be a starch and vegetable meal for which the body readily provides an alkaline environment, or a protein and vegetable meal, prompting the system to make an acid environment. Either way, your body will be able to extract all of the goodness and put it to use to replenish and repair your cells. You won't feel so sleepy after lunch because digesting the meal will not take all the energy from your body. You'll feel better because your body is not struggling with an impossible task. You will feel energized as your body is able to actually use the nutrients, which have been broken down and can be absorbed. In addition, you will not be poisoned by the fermentation by-products. For dinner, you can eat a meal of either starch or protein with vegetables. This makes for optimal digestion.

The common eating habits of our culture constantly create bad combinations for digestion. Most popular foods today are based on poor food combinations—spaghetti and meatballs, chicken stir-fry over rice, pizza, hamburgers on a bun with french fries, tacos, any sandwich that contains meat, and even trail mixes that combine protein nuts, starchy grains, and dried fruit. You can make better choices by following these four guidelines:

Eat starches with vegetables, *but not with protein or fruit (starches include grains, starchy vegetables such as potatoes, sweet potato, corn, legumes and beans, pasta, or bread).*

Eat protein with nonstarchy vegetables, *and not with starches (proteins include nuts, seeds, eggs, meat, or fish).*

Eat fruit alone. *Sweet fruits—such as bananas, dates, and grapes—should ideally be eaten after acid fruits, and acid fruits—such as citrus fruits, apples, mango, all berries, cherries, pears, apricots, and peaches—may be eaten with raw nuts).*

Melons should be eaten alone.

Why Fiber Is Important

Fiber is the indigestible portion of plant foods that nevertheless plays a vital role in human digestion. Soluble fiber produces food for the cells lining the gut and also supports friendly bacteria in the colon. Insoluble fiber aids in elimination, shortening the time it takes for the undigested food particles and toxins to pass through the intestinal tract. Both soluble and insoluble fiber help slow down the aging process by aiding the absorption of nutrients and the elimination of toxins. Although fiber is very important, it is lacking in our diets because we eat so much processed food and not enough fresh fruits and vegetables. Researchers recommend at least 30 grams of fiber per day, and many nutritional experts recommend 35 to 45 grams per day. The average American gets about 15 grams.

Fiber helps to normalize the body's insulin levels. In addition, fresh foods that are high in fiber are also high in nutrition, including the carotenes, flavonoids, and antioxidants that are known to be helpful in preventing and reversing premature aging. Good fiber sources include kidney beans, garbanzo beans, navy beans, gluten-free whole grains, legumes, and raw vegetables. As you work to reduce the amount of animal protein in your diet, increase the amount of these sources of plant protein. If you eat processed foods, get used to looking at the package label to find the fiber content.

Ready to Switch?

Every day, cellular machinery is being broken. However, as long as you have sufficient raw materials and good DNA blueprints to do repairs and build new cells, it's not a problem. *Problems arise because our poor diets and toxic overload prevent us from repairing all the damage.* DNA is being damaged constantly, in every cell. If damaged DNA is not repaired before the cell divides, the damage becomes permanent. The new cell will operate less efficiently because of the damage. As these less-efficient cells divide and make copies of themselves, and then become further damaged over time, your whole body will work less efficiently. *We call this aging.*

The Choice Is Simple

Human nutrition is extremely complex, but the choice that we need to make is simple. Either we continue to think of foods as entertainment and eat foods that make us sick, or we realize that food supplies essential raw materials for our cells and eat foods that make us healthy. Cells are chemical factories. More than 100,000 chemical reactions take place in each cell every second, producing thousands and thousands of chemicals that you need to stay alive and function. The raw materials for these chemical reactions come from the food you eat.

A chronic shortage of even one essential nutrient will affect the entire system and cause disease. This means you need to be mindful of everything you put into your mouth. Every mouthful should supply the maximum amount of nutrition, and we have to train ourselves to think about this. To get the nutrition we need, we have to eat real food. Real food is what nature provides, and it is loaded with nutrition. Unfortunately, real food is now in short supply; some people eat almost no real food at all. What they eat may be called "food," and may look like food to most people, but it is not fit to eat and it is making them sick. It is garbage. Modern processed foods are deficient in nutrients and high in toxins. Deficiency and toxicity are the two causes of disease, and modern processed foods cause both. This is why the Standard American Diet will not support healthy life—even in laboratory rats.

Richard's Story: Making the Choice

At six feet and 275 pounds, fifty-year-old Richard was obese and very concerned about his declining health. He was aging fast; he looked and felt much older than fifty. He got one cold after another, severe enough to cause him to miss work. He couldn't climb the stairs to his bedroom without huffing and puffing and feeling exhausted. He looked forward to leaving work and going home to rest. He was prediabetic, suffering from high triglycerides, low levels of "good" HDL cholesterol, high blood pressure, and insulin resistance. He suffered joint pain, back pain, muscle cramping, hair loss, skin problems, an enlarged prostate, and short-term memory loss. Richard ate the Standard American Diet that is full of calories but lacking essential nutrients, and he got little exercise. He was miserable, living a low-quality life.

After reading my book, *Never Be Sick Again,* Richard decided to implement what he learned to address his health problems. He never dreamed that improving his health would cause him to lose weight as well. Richard made the choice to cut the toxic Big Four out of his life (sugar, wheat, processed oils, and dairy/excess animal protein), and he added more fresh fruits, vegetables, whole grains, nuts and legumes. Richard worked to lower his toxic load by eating organic foods, eliminating processed foods and artificial sweeteners, and choosing nontoxic personal care products including shampoo, toothpaste, and deodorant. He asked me for recommendations on vitamins, and I explained that nutrients must be in the correct forms and ratios to optimize biological activity at the cellular level, and few supplements do this correctly. He began taking the supplements I recommended and quickly realized the vast difference in results between the supplements he had been taking and those specifically formulated to attain high biological activity. Richard also purchased a rebounder (mini-trampoline) that I recommended to help him exercise and improve his lymphatic drainage and detoxification.

Within months, Richard stopped getting colds, his energy soared, his memory improved, his aches and pains went away, and his skin became soft, smooth, and young looking. Within the first ten months, he lost fifty-six pounds. Life was less a chore and more fun. Richard's mood improved. As his health improved, he started walking to work, and now he even runs up the stairs. Richard's friends and coworkers are amazed at his miraculous transformation and can't believe how much more muscular, healthier, and younger he looks.

Richard made better choices, and it worked. Within two years, his weight was back to normal and his health problems had disappeared. He feels confident that he has found a permanent solution to his weight problem, and he now understands that normal weight and good health go together. Richard reports that he is feeling the best he has in his entire adult life. To achieve this, all he had to do was choose to give his cells what they need to do repairs and operate normally. By making these choices, he became healthier and biologically younger. He is once again enjoying life. Anyone can do this—including you—if you are willing to change some of your habits.

Fasting—The Closest We Get to a Biological Age Reset Button?

Fasting is a time-honored method of cleansing and rejuvenating the body. Fasting usually involves abstaining from some or all food for a period of time. When you fast, the amount of calories (energy) going into your body is significantly reduced.

In research laboratories, caloric restriction (usually by means of intermittent fasting) is the only intervention that consistently extends life span in a variety of species. Recent experiments also showed that intermittent fasting slowed down the rate of cell division and proliferation in mice. Because cell division affects both tumor growth and aging, the study's findings link fasting to both longer life and lower cancer risk.

A short (three- to seven-day) fast is a great way to start your new diet. Did you know that Eastern Orthodox monastic tradition prescribes a three-day fast at the start of Great Lent? The monks shut themselves up in their cells and abstain for three days from food and water. But you don't have to be that extreme. A fast with only vegetable juice works well to jump-start your body's detox pathways—and to prepare you for the adventure of eating and living the way you were designed.

Why Diets Fail

Whether what I am recommending here is earth-shattering news or not, the question is: Will you do it? The truth is that many knowledgeable and well-intentioned people struggle with making lasting changes to their diets until it's too late. Don't be one of them.

As we grow older, our need for nutrients generally increases, while our need for energy (calories) decreases. This makes it especially important that we carefully consider every bite we eat and *choose health every time.*

The anti-aging diet is not a fad diet. It's a permanent change in the way you eat and the way you think about food. All fad diets fail. Making a diet work for you is not a question of willpower, but rather a question of knowing what your body needs in order to restore itself to optimal health and stay biologically young. Most people's cells are already on a starvation diet, desperately missing essential nutrients and being overloaded with toxins. In order to sustain health, a diet needs to supply all the missing nutrients and support the body's natural detox process. A one-size diet doesn't fit all. Each one of us wakes up in the morning with a unique set of deficiencies and toxicities, as well as different caloric needs and lifestyle constraints. Cells have a grocery list, and it varies from one individual to the next and from one day to the next. That's why the important thing is to consistently choose nutrient-rich, whole, plant-based foods over the processed, disease-causing garbage that most people eat. When you eat the way you were designed to eat, your body gradually becomes your ally in choosing the right kind and quantity of food.

What is the best way to sabotage a great diet plan, gain unnecessary weight, and quadruple your junk-food cravings? Stress about it! Stress causes the body to release the hormone cortisol, which raises blood sugar, fueling the body for a fight-or-flight response. Over time, high stress leads to chronically elevated cortisol levels, driving appetite and weight gain. What's more, dieting stress leaves people more susceptible to the other stresses of everyday life, opening the door to binge or comfort eating that undoes any benefit of the diet itself.

So approach the anti-aging diet positively and creatively. Give yourself space to experiment and, yes, fail on occasion. Don't fault yourself for getting off track. Know that it will work for you, as it has for me and for countless thousands of others. Read more about coping with stress and maintaining a positive outlook in Chapter 6, "The Mental Pathway."

Supplements

Supplementation is now a necessity. In 1998 the National Academy of Sciences issued a report saying that *even if you eat a good diet, it is no longer possible to get all the nutrition you need for good health.* Here's the problem. While the human genome has survived almost unchanged since prehistoric times, the prehistoric diet has not. There is almost no place on the planet today where you can get the Paleolithic diet. Our soils are depleted of nutrients. The original varieties of many fruits and vegetables have become extinct. Our farmed animals are just as sick and nutrient deficient as the rest of the food chain. The reality is this: we simply cannot get all the nutrition we need from food alone, even if we eat a good diet with lots of fresh fruits and vegetables. We must supplement. People often ask what supplement they should take to slow down aging, but there is no one answer to this question. Vitamins and minerals work together synergistically. There is no one miracle anti-aging nutrient. We need every essential nutrient.

You Can No Longer Get All the Nutrition You Need from Food Alone

A key aspect of healthy eating is choosing foods that have not been adulterated. Eating foods that are as close as possible to their natural state is the only way to get the maximum amount of the nutrients that are found in fresh, raw foods. However, today's food supply is enormously compromised. The combination of modern chemical farming, harvesting before ripening, processing, pasteurizing, irradiating, storing, and shipping have all conspired to reduce the nutritional quality of our food to the point where it can no longer support healthy life. To begin with, farming with artificial fertilizers does not replace minerals in the soil. Additionally, pesticides and herbicides destroy beneficial bacteria and earthworms that transform inorganic minerals in the soil into organically available minerals that plants can take up into their roots. Mono-farming—planting the same crops year after year, without resting the field or rotating the crops—further depletes the soil. Our soils are now stripped of essential minerals, and if the minerals are not in the soil, they do not get into the plant. When you eat the plant, you don't get what you need.

Another reason modern produce is nutrient poor is the practice of harvesting crops before they are ripe. This helps get the food to you before it rots, but it reduces the nutritional content by up to 80 percent. This is because much of the nutrition develops in the last day or two of ripening. Then there is the problem of distribution. Food is best harvested when ripe and consumed shortly thereafter. With each passing hour after harvesting, nutrition is lost. It is significant that the average age of produce in the supermarket is two weeks, and some items are more than a year old. "Fresh" apples average about ten months old and are often more than a year old. They may still look like apples, but they have little nutritional value. Studies on "fresh" oranges have found that many contain no vitamin C whatsoever. These so-called fresh oranges are harvested green, stored in warehouses, artificially colored, and sold as fresh. In fact, the uniform color of nonorganic oranges is often due to the injection of an artificial dye into the skins—another reason to eat only organic oranges.

Food is remarkably hardy, but nutrients are not. Nutrients are easily lost or destroyed. For example, spinach loses 60 percent of its folic acid in three days. Vegetables such as asparagus, broccoli, and green beans lose 50 percent of their vitamin C before they reach the produce section. Cooking these vegetables will result in even more losses, including another 25 percent of the vitamin C, 70 percent of vitamin B_1, and 50 percent of B_2.

The nutritional content of every vegetable grown in the United States has undergone huge declines. A 2001 study in the *Nutrition Practitioner* looked at calcium levels in food over the period from 1940 to 1991. On average, in the space of fifty years, the calcium content of vegetables dropped by 46 percent—it is even less today. Consider a carrot. In order to get the same amount of calcium you got in one carrot half a century ago, you now have to eat two carrots. It would take four carrots to get the same magnesium, and up to twenty carrots to get the same amount of zinc. In 1940, one cup of spinach supplied 80 mg of iron. Today it would take 67 cups to get the same amount. Obviously, no one is eating all those extra vegetables.

Severe deficiencies of vitamins and minerals are uncommon in developed nations, but modest deficiencies are the norm. Maybe being short of one or two nutrients doesn't sound so bad to you, but remember this: To do its job of repairing your cells and keeping you biologically young, the body must have *everything* it needs. A chronic shortage of even one essential nutrient can throw the entire body out of balance. What happens when a tiny gear is missing from an expensive watch? No matter how expensive the watch, it will not keep good time. Consider a 2011 study in the *FASEB Journal,* finding that even moderate deficiencies of selenium and vitamin K impair normal cell functions that over time cause so-called age-related diseases.

Accelerated aging could even be viewed as a vitamin deficiency disease. Unfortunately, you simply cannot get anti-aging dosages of some vitamins and minerals, even if you eat a healthy, anti-aging diet. Although whole food should still be your main source of nutrition, supplementation is required to keep your cells from starvation. Vitamin and mineral supplements are essential and remarkably safe. But I'll be the first to admit that it is difficult to find brands that deliver high-quality, bioavailable nutrients. Nevertheless, it is possible to make them, and that is why I designed my own superior-quality Beyond Health brand supplements.

Your need for specific supplements will vary greatly according to your condition and your unique biochemistry. I will cover a few of the most common deficiencies and supplements in this chapter.

Multivitamins Make for Younger Cells

Taking a multivitamin is a good way to ensure that your body is getting a steady supply of essential nutrients, particularly if you've been eating poorly (which most of us are, despite what we believe) or if you have a health condition. Research supports the idea that multivitamins accelerate cell repairs and slow down aging. A 2009 study in the *American Journal of Clinical Nutrition* compared the biological age of the cells, as represented by length of telomeres, of those who took multivitamins and those who did not. Researchers found that taking a multivitamin every day adds about 5 percent of telomere length. Other studies have found the following nutrients to be very supportive of telomere length: vitamin B_{12}, vitamin D, omega-3 oils, zinc, vitamin C, and vitamin E.

As mentioned in Chapter 1, measuring telomeres is an advanced technique for determining the body's biological age. Telomeres— DNA sequences at the ends of chromosomes (like the plastic tips on shoelaces)—prevent "old" or damaged cells from replicating themselves indefinitely. As cells divide and accumulate DNA damage, the telomeres get shorter and shorter. Once the entire telomere is gone, the cell dies. As we age biologically, our repair deficits are reflected in lost telomere length. People with the shortest telomeres die years younger, and telomeres erode much faster in the presence of lots of free radicals and inflammation. This is why antioxidants extend life and protect against frailty.

CoQ_{10}

A coenzyme Q_{10} deficiency can lead to sluggish thinking and memory decline. People with high levels of CoQ_{10} have been proven in studies to have better motor abilities and higher mental acuity and energy. Supplementation is important because our ability to produce CoQ_{10} depletes as we age.

Zinc Boosts Immunity

Are you one of the 70 percent of Americans who, according to the USDA, aren't getting the Recommended Daily Intake (RDI) of zinc? Or could you be getting the RDI, but still not enough for optimal health?

Zinc is a key element in regulating cellular aging, but if you're not getting enough, accelerated aging is only one of a host of problems you're likely to face. Apart from its well-known role in immunity, zinc is required for the activity of more than 300 different enzymes and is involved in most major metabolic pathways. Here are just some of the reasons you may want to make sure you're getting enough zinc from food and supplements.

Immune Support. Zinc is crucial for thymus gland and T-cell function. According to a review of thirteen different studies by the Cochrane Collaboration, taking zinc within twenty-four hours of getting a cold can shorten the length of time you'll have the cold by one day as well as reduce severity of symptoms.

As we age, we need more zinc to maintain immunity, but our ability to absorb it decreases. As a result, zinc levels are often low among the elderly—possibly one of the main reasons aging is associated with a decline in immune system efficiency. According to a 2007 study sponsored by the National Institute of Aging, elderly nursing home residents who had normal levels of zinc were half as likely to get pneumonia as those who were deficient.

Cancer. Zinc has been shown to be protective against cancer. For example, in a 2011 study published in *Cancer Biology and Therapy,* zinc was found to suppress pancreatic cancer tumors. Other studies have found that zinc slows the development of prostate cancer.

Osteoporosis. Zinc is necessary for normal bone synthesis, and deficiency causes a reduction in osteoblast activity (osteoblasts are the cells that build new bone). Several studies have found that both older men and women with osteoporosis test low on zinc.

Skin. Zinc is used in treating acne, eczema, and other skin diseases. The University of Maryland Medical Center suggests taking 30 mg of zinc twice a day for a month to treat acne, and then reducing the dose to 30 mg daily. Zinc controls oil production in the skin and may control acne-related hormones.

Eyes. Zinc is the most abundant mineral in the eyes. It activates retinal dehydrogenase, an enzyme in the retina necessary for vision. Various studies have found zinc protective against macular degeneration and resulting vision loss.

Fertility. Both men and women need adequate zinc levels for reproduction, and it is often used to treat infertility. Zinc is involved in making sperm and is an important constituent in semen. In women, zinc is required for cell division and cell growth in the developing fetus.

The Senses. Two symptoms of zinc deficiency are diminished taste acuity and diminished sense of smell.

Zinc is highest in the protein-rich foods, particularly shellfish (especially oysters), but also in meat, poultry, and liver. Additional good sources of zinc are pumpkin and sunflower seeds, pecans, oats, and eggs. To maintain top immunity, 30 mg of zinc a day is recommended.

Magnesium: One of the Hardest-Working Minerals in the Body

Magnesium deficiency is associated with most "old age" diseases, including arthritis, Alzheimer's, cancer, diabetes, stroke, heart disease, hypertension, osteoporosis, insomnia, and thyroid disorders. Telomerase is an enzyme that repairs telomeres, but telomerase synthesis is dependent on the amount of magnesium available. So a shortage of magnesium will result in telomere shortening and aging.

The fourth most abundant mineral in the body, magnesium is involved in more than 300 types of biochemical reactions in the body. It helps maintain normal muscle and nerve function, keeps heart rhythm steady, supports a healthy immune system, and keeps bones strong. Magnesium also helps to regulate blood sugar levels, promote normal blood pressure, and support energy production and protein synthesis.

Any shortage of magnesium will result in multiple dysfunctions and so-called diseases. Magnesium is absolutely essential to oxygen respiration. It is involved in every single step in the production of energy in normal cells. Yet most of us are deficient in this mineral, and that causes cells to switch energy production to fermentation, which produces much less energy, more acid, and lots of dangerous free radicals. About 70 percent of Americans do not consume the recommended daily intake of magnesium, and more than 80 percent of our elderly do not. Older adults are at a particular risk for magnesium deficiency. In aged individuals, magnesium absorption decreases and renal excretion of magnesium increases. Older adults are also more likely to be taking drugs that interact with magnesium. Virtually everyone should be taking a high-quality magnesium supplement.

Magnesium is not very easily absorbed by the digestive tract. According to Sally Fallon Morell in *Nourishing Traditions,* only about 50 percent of magnesium in foods is absorbed. If you have digestive problems, such as a leaky gut and food allergies, you may not be absorbing even that much. Even people with a healthy gut who eat a balanced high-magnesium diet with magnesium-rich vegetables, whole grains, nuts, and seeds may not be able to rely upon food alone to provide sufficient magnesium because our soils are so depleted. Mercury fillings and other forms of exposure to mercury prevent magnesium from being absorbed and utilized by the body. Fluoride also binds with magnesium and prevents absorption.

Dietary fat can also interfere with magnesium absorption, as does vitamin D deficiency. Eating a lot of dairy products and other foods high in calcium can also affect magnesium levels. Drinking caffeine, carbonated soft drinks, and alcohol wastes magnesium. So does eating sugar. Cocoa is a good source of magnesium, but it is rarely if ever eaten without sugar, which depletes magnesium. There are also a number of drugs that interfere with magnesium absorption and utilization, including the birth control pill, antibiotics, antihistamines, and aspirin. Last but not least, stress uses a lot of magnesium. If you are under stress, you need more magnesium.

Selenium Protects the Brain

Certain essential proteins, such as the powerful antioxidant enzyme glutathione peroxidase, are dependent on selenium. When selenium is in short supply, the lack of this critical enzyme results in cancer, heart disease, arthritis, aging, and loss of immune and brain functioning.

Selenium helps protect the brain from aging. There is a lot of mercury in our environment, and a toxic form of mercury, methylmercury, accumulates in the brain. Methylmercury damages the brain and nervous system, contributing to the aging process. Selenium helps to neutralize methylmercury, and supplementation is usually needed. Selenium blood levels typically drop by 7 percent after age sixty and 24 percent after age seventy-five.

B Vitamins Reverse Aging

The benefits of B vitamins are truly amazing. B vitamins work together as a team and are essential to a multitude of functions in the body, including energy production. This is why it is important to be sure you are getting the whole team. As you age, the need for B vitamins increases. Muscles start to deteriorate after age thirty, but a combination of regular exercise and B vitamins can actually reverse this process. Vitamin B_6 is important for healthy brain function and mental clarity. Vitamin B_3 is critical for maintaining the body's energy levels. Vitamin B_{12} slows down telomere degradation, and B_{12} supplementation has been associated with increased telomere length. A B_{12} deficiency can cause symptoms of aging, including cognitive problems and poor memory, muscle weakness, fatigue, shakiness, unsteady gait, low blood pressure, mood disorders, and depression. A high-quality multivitamin can supply what most people need, but most B_{12} supplements are in the form of cyanocobalamin, a biologically inappropriate form of B_{12}.

Vitamin C: The King of Vitamins

Vitamin C is one of the most powerful vitamins you can take. It retards telomere shortening, slowing the aging process. Most people don't get enough of this youth-enhancing, anti-aging vitamin that stabilizes blood pressure, boosts the immune system, fights colds and flu, and is an outstanding cancer fighter. It is a powerful anti-oxidant that neutralizes free radicals produced in the body. It is also necessary for synthesizing collagen, the most important protein for maintaining elasticity and strength of the skin, arteries, and other body tissues. Vitamin C is your best defense against wrinkles. Supplement with 6,000 mg per day in divided doses.

Vitamin D: A Fitness Booster for Older Adults

Vitamin D significantly increases the production of telomerase, the enzyme that repairs telomeres. This helps to keep your telomeres long, slows aging, and keeps you biologically young.

Vitamin D plays an important role in muscle function, and low levels reduce muscle strength and physical performance. According to data from the National Institute on Aging, older adults who have trouble walking several blocks or climbing a flight of stairs may be deficient in vitamin D. Low vitamin D levels have also been linked to diabetes, hypertension, cardiovascular disease, and lung disease—conditions that frequently cause decline in physical function.

About one-third of older adults are short of vitamin D. It's difficult to get enough vitamin D through diet alone. The best source is exposure to sunlight, and if you do not spend enough time outdoors, you may need to supplement with vitamin D. Current recommendations are that people older than seventy get 800 IU of vitamin D per day. However, many researchers believe that to be too low and recommend 5,000 to 10,000 IU per day. It is easy to measure vitamin D with a blood test, and you should keep your vitamin D level at the upper end of the normal range—above 50 ng/ml.

Vitamin E: A Powerful Antioxidant

Vitamin E fights aging by protecting against oxidative damage to tissues. It retards telomere shortening, thus slowing the aging process. A powerful antioxidant, vitamin E helps prevent cellular aging by neutralizing free radicals that can lead to genetic mutations and tissue damage. Supplement with 400 to 800 IU per day. Vitamin E has been extensively studied, and 800 IU per day will slash LDL oxidation by 40 percent and improve immune function.

Acetyl L-Carnitine and Lipoic Acid

Damage to mitochondria (the energy-producing powerhouses of the cell) is a major contributor to aging and associated degenerative diseases. Lipoic acid is a powerful antioxidant compound that offers protection from age-related memory decline and strokes. Acetyl L-carnitine transports fatty acid fuel into the mitochondria, supporting normal oxygen respiration in the cell. The two working together synergistically appear to reverse much of the decay process due to aging and to improve brain and other functions by rejuvenating the mitochondria.

Curcumin

Curcumin is a component of the spice turmeric. It works well for the many conditions that are driven by inflammation and also reduces edema. It lowers cholesterol and triglyceride levels, helps to prevent heart disease by inhibiting inflammation and oxidative damage, and prevents blood clots by inhibiting platelet aggregation. Curcumin can stop the buildup of the destructive beta-amyloid protein in the brain. Alzheimer's rates in India are among the lowest in the world, and research shows that curcumin is responsible.

Supplementation Is Essential

Vitamin and mineral deficiencies are a critical problem. Nobel Prize winner Dr. Linus Pauling once said, "You can trace every sickness, every disease, and every ailment to a mineral deficiency." Yet the mineral content of our farm soils has decreased dramatically in the last hundred years. Combine that with the mineral losses from food processing, and the result is that almost every American is mineral-deficient to one degree or another. No wonder more than three out of four Americans have a diagnosable chronic disease. You may have no symptoms, but if you consume foods that have little nutritional value or are toxic, you are almost certainly in the early stages of disease. The only way out of disease is to eat fresh, whole foods and supplement with high-quality supplements.

The Bottom Line

✓ Cell damage occurs all the time. Every day, billions of your cells divide to create new cells, and if the damage is not repaired before cell division, the damage becomes permanent. Your new cells will operate less efficiently, and as this process is repeated, aging occurs.

✓ A key to staying biologically young is to provide your body with sufficient raw materials (nutrients) every day to make repairs and create healthy new cells.

✓ The foundation of a nutrient-rich, anti-aging diet is raw, fresh, preferably organic vegetables, including sprouts. This can be augmented with a moderate amount of fruit (avoid fruit juices), moderate amounts of soaked raw nuts and seeds, healthy oils, legumes and small portions of high-quality animal protein. Non-gluten grains may also be eaten in moderation, and eight glasses of pure water a day are recommended.

✓ At least 80 percent of your diet should be raw, in the form of salads, vegetable juices, and blenderized drinks. Cooking robs foods of nutrients, destroys enzymes, and adds toxins. The higher the temperature and the longer the cooking time, the more damage is done.

✓ Without good digestion, nutrients from foods do not get absorbed, and undigested food promotes the creation of dangerous toxins. Take time to chew your food well and use the rules for proper food combining to optimize digestion.

✓ Dietary fiber is needed for eliminating toxins. Although the average American gets about 15 grams of fiber daily, 30–45 grams have been recommended.

✓ Intermittent fasting has been shown to slow the aging process and increase lifespan. A three- to seven-day vegetable juice fast is a good way to begin your anti-aging diet.

✓ Even the best diet today does not supply adequate nutrients; nutritional supplements have become a necessity.

✓ Nutrients act as a team, and all the vitamins and minerals are necessary. A chronic deficiency of even one nutrient will affect the entire system and lead to aging and disease. A high-quality multivitamin-mineral is the foundation of a good anti-aging supplement program.

✓ As we age, our need for nutrients goes up, while our ability to absorb them and our need for calories go down. Zinc, magnesium, and selenium are the minerals most likely to be deficient. We also need to take care to get adequate B vitamins, and vitamins C, D, and E. CoQ_{10} and acetyl-L-carnitine levels decline with age, and supplementation is recommended over the age of fifty. Additional anti-aging supplements are lipoic acid, curcumin, the carotenes, garlic, silymarin, ginkgo, and Beyond Health's Age Defense Formula.

✓ Although severe nutrient deficiencies in developed countries are rare, moderate deficiencies are the norm. Virtually every American is deficient in at least several nutrients. If you are one of them, even though you don't yet have symptoms, you are almost certainly in the early stages of disease and accelerated aging.

CHAPTER 5

The Toxin Pathway

Aging is a slow poisoning,
a lifetime accumulation of
toxins in the body.

—Mirika von Viczay, ND, PhD

As the first generation of man
exposed to an unprecedented plethora of
daily chemicals, we have learned that stored
chemicals can mimic any disease.
"Incurable" chronic diseases that were thought
to have no known cause often disappear
when toxic chemicals are gone.

—Sherry Rogers, MD, author of *Tired or Toxic?*

"**E**VERYBODY IN THIS COUNTRY needs to be detoxified because we've all become 'toxic dumpsites,'" said Doris J. Rapp, MD, past president of the American Academy of Environmental Medicine in her book *Our Toxic World: A Wake-Up Call.* Toxicity is one of the two causes of all disease, and it is largely responsible for our epidemic of chronic disease and accelerated aging.

Toxic Planet, Toxic People

If we eat good food and drink clean water, are we basically okay? For most of us, the answer is no. We live in a toxic world where we are accumulating toxins faster than we can get rid of them. Our bodies are constantly interacting with our immediate and distant environments. The air we breathe, the foods we eat, the water we drink, and even the lotions we put on our skin all introduce foreign substances that affect our body chemistry and lower our resistance to disease. The problem is that each year our world is becoming more toxic. Newly invented chemicals constantly enter our lives and accumulate in our tissues. Annoying symptoms like headaches, insomnia, gastrointestinal disturbances, joint and muscle pain, allergies, increased pulse rate, and high blood pressure—and serious debilitating conditions like heart disease, cancer, immune disorders, endocrine disorders, and many more—can result from these chemical exposures. Many environmental toxins disrupt neurotransmitters in the brain and the nervous system, giving rise to anxiety, depression, fatigue, and hyperactivity. They also drive disorders like Alzheimer's, Parkinson's, and autism.

Multiple Chemical Sensitivity Syndrome: Robin's Story

Toxins are now causing an enormous amount of disease in our society, including entirely new disease syndromes that bewilder our physicians, such as chemical sensitivity, chronic fatigue, and fibromyalgia. The problem is our physicians have not been trained to look for the causes of the problems they see in their patients. Also, many toxins are difficult to see, smell, or taste, and can affect us even in exceedingly small concentrations, so it is hard to believe that something nearly imperceptible could do so much damage. It is the cumulative and synergistic effect of our constant exposure to the tens of thousands of man-made chemicals in our environment that is exceeding our capacity to cope with these toxins. One of the results of this overload is a disorder called Chemical Sensitivity Syndrome. This syndrome is something I know a lot about, since my own case was as extreme as any ever recorded.

In many ways, Robin was a typical case. In her mid-thirties, she started experiencing food and pollen allergies, and became sensitive to chemical odors, such as those in the detergent aisle of the supermarket. Robin became pregnant, and immediately after the birth of her child, her body crashed. She developed debilitating chemical sensitivities, along with chronic fatigue, asthma, frequent headaches, hypoglycemia, frequent infections, digestive problems, and hypothyroidism.

Like myself, Robin became a universal reactor, suffering debilitating reactions to common foods and chemical odors—she was reacting to everything in her environment. She suffered anaphylactic reactions daily and passed out several times a day. Robin was unable to do any meaningful work, not even to care for her children. Robin went to more than twenty physicians, only to get sicker and sicker. (I went to thirty-six medical doctors and ended up almost dying from the toxic drugs they prescribed.) Conventional physicians don't understand disease, so all they do is attempt to suppress symptoms with toxic drugs. Since Robin was already in toxic overload, the additional toxic load of the drugs made her much sicker. Robin finally found a holistic physician. His first recommendation was to read my book *Never Be Sick Again*. Robin read the book and then called asking for advice.

The recommendation I gave Robin was simple. Give her cells what they need and keep them free of what they don't need. Robin started to take regular saunas to detoxify her body. She removed the toxic Big Four from her diet, started eating more fresh fruits and vegetables, and started on a supplement program that I recommended. She also rebounded to get the movement she needed to help supply nutrients to her cells and to remove toxins. Robin also cleaned up her environment. She got rid of the synthetic fiber carpets in her home, and replaced them with carpets made from natural fiber. She discarded a new mattress that was outgassing dozens of toxic chemicals, including flame retardants, which were poisoning her as she slept. She helped to detoxify her home with help from National Allergy Supply (see Appendix C).

By including more high-quality organic foods in her diet and removing the deadly Big Four, getting on a good supplement program, and actively detoxifying, Robin was able to get most of her life back within a year. Within three years, she was able to return to work. Robin and I agree that living through such an experience changed our lives forever. I decided to devote the remainder of my life to teaching people everywhere how to get well and stay well, and Robin decided to bring environmental information into schools. Robin formed a Massachusetts nonprofit called Green Schools. Green Schools has interacted with more than 200 schools in New England, and even more around the world, helping them to create a healthier environment for children. (See Appendix C for more information about Green Schools.)

We all need to realize that we live in a toxic world. These toxins are affecting us, some more than others, and there is no question that toxins play a substantial role in accelerated aging. Fortunately, almost anyone can reduce their toxic exposure, simply and inexpensively, by following the suggestions in this chapter.

What Are Toxins?

Any substance that causes a cell to malfunction is a toxin. Malfunctioning cells will manifest as some form of disease or aging, but the root cause is whatever is disrupting the normal cell function. Even water can act as a toxin if too much gets into a cell. Almost all man-made chemicals have a toxic effect on the body.

How Toxins Work

Toxins can harm us in numerous ways by interfering with the body's internal communication and its ability to regulate and repair itself, or by impairing its ability to create energy. Energy is life—without energy, nothing happens, and less energy means less repair. Toxins impair oxygen respiration and the ability of cells to create the energy of life. For example, heavy metals like lead and mercury shut down enzymes that cells need to produce critical, life-sustaining molecules, such as the high-energy compounds produced through oxygen respiration. We all have too much lead and mercury in our bodies. Industrial chemicals like PCBs, BPA, and phthalates are xenoestrogens that mimic the body's own hormones and give false signals to cells and genes, causing them to malfunction. Some toxins inhibit cell-to-cell communication, interfering with the body's ability to self-regulate. Some toxins directly damage DNA, causing mutations, while others interact with DNA and change how genes express. Other toxins damage immunity or interfere with oxygen transport. Even very small amounts of toxins can be devastating to health and contribute to premature aging. Unfortunately, due to our poor diets, our ability to handle toxins is declining, while our exposure is growing on an unprecedented scale.

We Live in a Sea of Toxins

For the last century, mankind has been unwittingly involved in a vast chemistry experiment. We now know that chemical living is having a catastrophic effect on our health, yet it is not only continuing—it's expanding. We don't realize how many toxins bombard us every minute of every day because we can't see them. They are in the air we breathe, the water we drink, and the food we eat. They are in our toothpaste, shampoo, cosmetics, cars, clothes, newspapers, magazines, furniture, and the prescription and over-the-counter drugs we take. More than 3,000 chemicals are added to our food. More than 700 industrial pollutants have been found in city drinking water. One billion pounds of pesticides are used in the United States every year, and a percentage of that ends up in our bodies. Our oceans and waterways are so contaminated that it is now unsafe to eat more than a small quantity of fish. These chemicals affect every cell in your body and most of your exposure occurs without your knowledge—which is why you need to educate yourself.

Did you know that, according to the 2008–2009 Report of the President's Cancer Panel, less than 10 percent of the nearly 80,000 chemicals used in commerce today have been tested for their capacity to damage your health? We are told that our exposure to each chemical is very small, and in general, this is true. However, when you add up all the small amounts of the thousands of toxins we encounter daily, the exposure is significant. According to scientists at the United Nations Educational, Scientific, and Cultural Organization (UNESCO), our combined exposure to industrial pollutants can be as much as seventy-five times the dose considered toxic in animals. Consider that many of these chemicals build up in your tissues year after year, and you begin to see why you must be proactive and protect yourself as much as you can.

Exceeding Our Capacity

Why is chemical living so dangerous to our health? It is a basic principle in biology that organisms function best when they eat the food and live in the environment to which they are adapted by their evolution. We have fundamentally changed both our food and our environment, making them toxic to our cells. Our body has a built-in capacity to protect and detoxify itself. However, our chemical exposure is such that most of us have exceeded that capacity. Worse, these toxins have damaged our detoxification pathways, and our poor nutrition further inhibits these pathways. The result is that we are accumulating toxins in our tissues faster than we can get rid of them.

Our genes evolved 100,000 years before the petroleum age, which began only a century ago. Since then, our environment has become a sea of petroleum-based, oil-soluble toxins, most of which did not even exist before World War II. Never before exposed to these chemicals, nature did not design a way for us to get rid of them. Our detoxification systems don't have a solution to a problem that didn't exist when our genes evolved. As a result, the average person is bioaccumulating between 300 and 500 man-made chemicals. For example, styrene from plastic drinking cups and food packaging is now found in almost 100 percent of human tissue in America. PCBs, dioxins, paradichlorobenzene (in mothballs and deodorizers), sodium lauryl sulfate (in soap, shampoo, and toothpaste), triclosan (in antibacterial soap and underarm deodorants), and many others are piling up in our tissues. Many of these chemicals are known carcinogens and hormone disruptors.

Human fat cells make hormones, and now those same fat cells are bioaccumulating hormone disruptors. No wonder so many of us have hormonal abnormalities and our children are entering puberty at younger and younger ages.

Virtually all Americans are in toxic overload. *A major reason we get sicker as we get older is that we progressively become more toxic.* We are now one of the most polluted species on the planet. Human flesh is so contaminated it would not pass the USDA food safety standards!

In 2009, the CDC published its Fourth National Report on Human Exposure to Environmental Chemicals. This report listed 212 compounds that were found in the blood and urine of most Americans. Six chemicals appeared in virtually every person:

Polybrominated diphenyl ethers (PBDEs)

Bisphenol-A (BPA)

Perfluorooctanoic acid (PFOA)

Acrylamide

Mercury

Methyl tert-butyl ether (MTBE)

Each of these is known to be highly dangerous to your health. Here's why and what you can do to protect yourself.

Polybrominated Diphenyl Ethers (PBDEs)

PBDEs are used as flame retardants. These chemicals are added to many consumer products, including furniture, mattresses, carpeting, and computers. They build up in human fat tissue, causing damage to the nervous system, liver, and kidneys. PBDEs have also been linked to sexual dysfunction, thyroid problems, brain disorders, and cancer.

American women's breast milk has the highest PBDE levels in the world. Before purchasing carpets, mattresses, and upholstered furniture, check to see if they have been treated with flame retardants. If so, try to find nontoxic substitutes.

Bisphenol-A (BPA)

Bisphenol-A (BPA) is found in plastics, including polycarbonate water bottles and epoxy can linings. About 85 percent of all food and beverage cans sold in the United States have plastic linings that will leach out BPA. Another important source of BPA is cash register and credit card receipts—BPA is used to make this special kind of paper. *BPA is toxic at exceedingly low concentrations.* It is an endocrine disruptor that can mimic the body's own hormones and unbalance the entire hormone system. It has been linked to heart disease, diabetes, sexual dysfunction, immune dysfunction, behavioral disorders, asthma, obesity, liver damage, DNA damage, and cancer. BPA alters the expression of genes. Children can inherit this change from their parents and even pass it on to their children. It is scary to think that even if we ban a toxic chemical like BPA, the epigenetic change (environmental alteration of gene expression) may remain encoded in our genes for generations.

Avoid using plastic water bottles and do not consume canned foods or beverages. Minimize your handling of receipts. Consider keeping them in a small plastic bag rather than in your wallet, and don't throw them into your recycle bin. Traces of BPA have been showing up in all kinds of recycled products, from mailing envelopes to toilet paper. Be aware that many products labeled "BPA-Free" contain chemical alternatives such as BPS, which may not be any safer.

Perfluorooctanoic Acid (PFOA)

Perfluorooctanoic acid (PFOA) is used in nonstick cookware, stain-resistant clothing, certain food packaging, and heat-resistant products. Limit your use of such products. Studies verify that PFOA contributes to liver and immune system dysfunction, as well as infertility, other reproductive problems, and cancer.

Acrylamide

Acrylamide is formed when frying, roasting, grilling, or baking carbohydrate-rich foods at temperatures above 120 degrees centigrade (248 degrees Fahrenheit). A number of foods, such as fried chicken, bread, chips, French fries, and even coffee contain acrylamide. Tobacco smoking also generates substantial amounts of acrylamide. Acrylamide is known to cause cancer. Avoid acrylamide-containing foods.

Mercury

Mercury is one of the most toxic metals known. Yet it is found in virtually every American, causing harm even in extremely small amounts. The principal sources are silver dental fillings, vaccinations, and fish. Mercury damages DNA and disables enzymes needed for oxygen respiration. Mercury cuts the oxygen-carrying capacity of the blood in half and lowers immunity. It impairs enzymes needed to produce energy through oxygen respiration, shifting energy production to fermentation. Studies have shown that removing mercury fillings from your mouth can result in a 50 to 300 percent increase in T-cell (immune cell) counts. In fact, white cell abnormalities, such as those observed in leukemia, have disappeared when mercury amalgam fillings were removed. Elevated levels of mercury and other toxic metals, such as lead, cadmium, and arsenic, shut down our resistance to aging and disease. When dealing with chronic disease, get tested for heavy metal contamination and remove these from your body.

Methyl Tert-Butyl Ether (MTBE)

Methyl tert-butyl ether (MTBE) is a gasoline additive. It was supposed to make gasoline burn cleaner and help reduce air pollution. Instead it poisoned our water supply, and most states have banned its use because it causes neurological and reproductive problems. Unfortunately, it is a persistent chemical, and it is still polluting our water supplies, as well as most Americans' bodies. Another source of MTBE is cigarette smoke.

Hundreds of chemicals like MTBE have been found in the cord blood of newborns. We are poisoning our babies! Today's mothers are so toxic, children are born loaded with toxins. These chemicals are known to cause birth defects, abnormal development, damage to the brain and nervous system, and cancer. Research shows that children born with the highest amounts of chemicals in their bodies have lower IQs, more behavioral problems, and suffer more chronic disease, both as children and as adults. It is imperative that women who are planning to have children avoid toxins and engage in proactive detoxification to lower the toxic load in their bodies.

Toxicity and Aging

By retirement age, our accumulated toxic loads are more than sufficient to cause chronic disease. At the same time, the detoxification capacity of our kidneys and liver diminishes with age. Add to that the toxic burden of multiple prescription drugs, and what you have is fatigue, poor memory, disorientation, and accelerated aging in our older population.

Virtually every chronic disease has been associated with certain toxins. For example, diabetes has been linked to arsenic in drinking water. Alzheimer's has been associated with environmental mercury and aluminum. Automotive pollution increases the risk of stroke. Excess lead, copper, iron, and mercury all contribute to arthritis.

Iron Toxicity Causes Aging

The body needs iron, but the difference between too much and too little is small. So it is easy to get too much. Iron toxicity has been linked to diabetes, heart disease, arthritis, Alzheimer's disease, and cancer. It is far more common and dangerous than many people realize. The standard American diet includes excess iron because of high consumption of red meat and because iron is added to most white flour products. Plus, many supplements, over-the-counter preparations, and prescription drugs contain iron.

How does excess iron damage your health? One way is by disabling enzymes. Excess iron displaces essential minerals such as copper, manganese, zinc, and others in enzyme-binding sites. This causes the enzymes to malfunction, which damages your metabolic machinery and results in cellular malfunction, aging, and disease. In addition, excess iron causes inflammation, resulting in aging and disease.

Excess Aluminum Causes Alzheimer's

Aluminum is a well-known neurotoxin. Several aluminum-containing compounds have the ability to cross the brain-blood barrier and produce pathological changes, eventually leading to Alzheimer's. Aluminum damages the brain by displacing vital minerals in enzymes and proteins. To reduce your exposure to aluminum, do not drink most tap water or anything in aluminum cans. Do not use aluminum-containing antacids or deodorants. Do not cook in aluminum pots and pans, and do not cook or store your foods in aluminum foil. Supplement with calcium, magnesium, and zinc.

Toxins Cause Deficiency

Toxins also cause nutrient deficiency. Our exposure to toxins is placing an unprecedented burden on our bodies. Every molecule that gets into the body has to be metabolized in some way. Beneficial molecules, such as nutrients, "pay for themselves," as the body is able to recover the energy expended during metabolism. Toxins, on the other hand, are "pure expense." Processing toxic molecules dramatically increases our need for nutrients, particularly antioxidants. Our need for antioxidants more than tripled in the twenty-year period from 1970 to 1990, and it is undoubtedly even higher today. Meanwhile, in the same period, the antioxidant levels in foods dropped to less than half. The deadly combination of toxic overload and poor diet acting together is directly responsible for our epidemic of chronic disease and premature aging, as well as the many mystery illnesses, such as chemical sensitivity syndrome and chronic fatigue syndrome. (A syndrome is a collection of symptoms for which conventional medicine cannot find a specific cause.) All are products of the late twentieth century. Fortunately, all these can be corrected with real food, supplements, exercise, and protecting yourself from toxins. Here's how.

What Can You Do About Toxins?

The body is able to cope with toxins up to a certain point—then you get sick. Some researchers believe we have already crossed the line and may have compromised all future life on the planet. As bad as things are, there are actions each of us can take to reduce the impact of toxins on our health. Here is what to do:

Reduce your daily exposure to toxins.
Nutritionally support your detoxification systems.
Remove stored toxins from your body.

If you do these three things well, your body will no longer be in toxic overload and will have the opportunity to function normally.

Remember, accelerated aging is a disease. All you need to stay biologically young is to be healthy. Health is created when all the exquisitely complex metabolic machinery inside your cells is operating normally. While this is happening, you cannot be sick. We get old and sick by failing to supply the nutrients our cells need and by introducing toxins into the system.

Reduce Daily Exposure

To get well or stay well, you must learn how to reduce your daily exposure to toxins. You need to determine the sources of your exposure and avoid them as best you can, so you can lower your total toxic load. You can't save a sinking ship if water is coming in faster than you are pumping it out. About 80 percent of your toxic exposure is under your personal control to avoid. By exercising this control, you can reduce your toxic load enough that your body can safely detoxify the remainder. All you have to do is make better choices about the foods you eat, the air you breathe, the water you drink, and the products you purchase.

Toxins in Our Food

To reduce your toxic exposure, start with the foods you eat. Toxins get into our food through pesticides, chemical fertilizers, environmental pollution, processing, and packaging. According to the USDA, more than 70 percent of fruits and vegetables contain pesticide residues. There are also naturally occurring toxins in plants and environmental toxins that bioaccumulate in animals. To one degree or another, almost the entire food supply has been poisoned; there is little available at a supermarket that is not toxic in some way.

The question you need to ask yourself is: How much gunk can you put in your cells before they get really screwed up and make you sick and old? In some cases, it doesn't take much. The combined effects of multiple pesticides can magnify by thousands of times the effect of any one of them acting alone. As much as possible, avoid processed foods and eat only fresh, organically grown foods. Do not use pesticides in your home or garden. There are many safe alternatives. If you need an insecticide, use a safe, natural product like Orange Guard.

Eat Organic

Does it really make a difference if you eat organic? A 2003 study in *Environmental Health Perspectives* fed one group of children a 75 percent organic diet while another group was fed 75 percent conventional foods. The children's urine was measured for pesticides. The children eating conventional foods measured four times higher than the official safety limit. Yet, after only a few days of being on a mostly organic diet, the children in the second group measured only one-sixth as much as the conventional group and within the safety limit. *Eating organic makes a big difference!*

Meat, dairy products, and fish are contaminated with a variety of toxins, including insecticides, fungicides, weed killers, hormones, antibiotics, prescription drugs, industrial chemicals, PCBs, dioxins, flame retardants, and heavy metals. The United States is the world's largest user of pesticides. People who work with pesticides—farmers, pesticide applicators, manufacturers, and crop dusters—have high rates of all kinds of cancers and other chronic diseases. By eating only organic eggs and meat and cutting out dairy entirely, you can eliminate up to 80 percent of your exposure to some of the most harmful toxins. Far from being an impossible task, protecting yourself from toxins in your food is within reach when you can achieve an 80 percent reduction so easily.

When Organic Is Not an Option

The safest bet is to always buy organic. When eating nonorganic produce, it's good to know which are the least contaminated. Following is a list of conventional produce that tested with the lowest pesticide residues:

asparagus	grapefruit	peas
avocados	kiwi	pineapple
bananas	mangoes	plums
blueberries	melons	radishes
broccoli	mushrooms	tangerines
cabbage	onions	tomatoes
cauliflower	oranges	watermelons
eggplant	papaya	

On the other hand, these fruits and vegetables are sprayed the most. Buy organic only:

apples	lettuce	pumpkin
celery	nectarines	raspberries
cherries	peaches	spinach
cucumbers	pears	squash
grapes	peppers	strawberries
green beans	potatoes	

Eliminate All Processed Foods

It is best to eliminate all processed foods. Not only are they deficient in nutrition, but virtually all of them are contaminated with toxins. Dairy, meats, and farmed salmon contain flame retardants. Milk is a toxic soup filled with pesticides, antibiotics, dioxins, hormones, sulfa drugs, tranquilizers, and other contaminants. Bread is often contaminated with potassium bromate, used as a dough conditioner. Bromate competes with iodine in the thyroid, causing thyroid malfunction. Commercial peanut butter is loaded with toxic chemical residues. According to the 1982–1986 Total Diet Study, conducted by the FDA, peanut butter had a whopping 183 residues, including highly carcinogenic aflatoxin, produced by a mold that grows on peanuts. Frozen french fries contained seventy different pesticide residues. Frozen pizzas had sixty-seven industrial chemicals and pesticides. Frozen chocolate cake contained sixty-one toxic residues, and milk chocolate had ninety-three. Advertisers never mention these facts when they write catchy jingles for processed foods.

Of special concern are processed meats. In 2007, the American Institute for Cancer Research reviewed more than 7,000 clinical studies examining the connection between diet and cancer and came to this conclusion: No amount of processed meat is safe, therefore no one should eat processed meats. Processed meats such as bacon, ham, hot dogs, pastrami, pepperoni, salami, and some sausages and hamburgers are preserved by salting, smoking, or adding chemical preservatives. Smoking creates polycyclic aromatic hydrocarbons, carcinogens that contaminate the meat. Nitrites, added to preserve the meat from bacteria and discoloration, are metabolized into nitrosamines that are known to be carcinogenic.

Eliminate All Genetically Modified Foods

Genetically modified foods pose numerous health risks. Many GMO crops are engineered either to produce their own insecticides or to tolerate high doses of externally applied pesticides. People who eat these crops ingest insecticides that are known to damage human cells as well as insect cells. These dangerous insecticides have even been found in the blood of pregnant women. The practice of leaving plant material on the field until the next season is polluting streams, groundwater, wells, and springs. As a practical matter, avoiding GMO foods means you will need to eliminate all corn and soy from your diet. Virtually all of the corn and soy grown in the United States is genetically modified. Even organic varieties may have been inadvertently cross-pollinated with genetically modified crops in neighboring fields.

The Problem with Arsenic

Arsenic is highly toxic and directly contributes to aging. It is a carcinogen and a hormone disruptor, affecting every bodily system. Arsenic binds to enzymes and other molecules, disrupting their function in the body. It also induces DNA-damaging free radicals. It is particularly dangerous to older adults, because DNA's ability to repair itself declines with age. In addition to accelerated aging, people with elevated arsenic are more likely to experience depression, high blood pressure, and circulatory problems, which all too often result in bypass surgery.

Arsenic is present in most fluoridated tap water. It is used in pressure-treated wood, pharmaceuticals, poultry feed, and pesticides. It is also found in groundwater. Many people consider brown rice syrup a healthy alternative to sugar, but brown rice syrup contains high levels of arsenic. As it grows, rice absorbs arsenic from the soil, more so than other plants. Brown rice and brown rice syrup contain more arsenic than white rice and rice starch because arsenic concentrates in the brown hull. This problem extends to organically farmed rice, because even organic rice soaks up arsenic already present in the soil. Watch out for gluten-free products made with rice flour and foods sweetened with brown rice syrup. As Americans opt for more rice-containing foods, promoted as healthy alternatives to conventional processed foods, they're unknowingly ingesting more arsenic.

Packaging Matters

Packaging materials (such as plastic wrap, plastic bottles, milk containers, juice boxes, Styrofoam, and epoxy can linings) can leach toxins into our foods before we eat them. Portions of the polymers, plasticizers, stabilizers, fillers, and even colorants in plastic wrap can dissolve into the food, so avoid foods packaged in plastic. Choose more appropriate materials, such as paper and glass—or buy in bulk. Even the wax paper used to package breakfast cereals has been found to leach toxic chemicals into the cereal. Why purchase organic meat in a Styrofoam tray topped with plastic shrink-wrap or organic canned goods in an epoxy-lined can? To avoid the contaminants, you need to know about every aspect of the foods you eat, including the safety of their packaging.

Use the Right Cookware

The pots and pans you use for cooking interact with your food and introduce some level of toxins into the food. The safest choices are ceramic or glass, such as CorningWare and Pyrex, as well as ceramic enameled cookware. Stainless steel contains nickel, a known toxin. A study in the *Journal of the American Dietetic Association* found that toxic chemicals from stainless steel pots, including nickel, iron, and chromium, enter food during cooking. That being said, stainless can still be a better choice than other alternatives such as aluminum. Aluminum—from pots, pans, and aluminum foil—is a toxic contaminant that has been linked to Alzheimer's, rheumatism, migraines, and other problems. Cast iron leaches iron into food. Too much iron rapidly accelerates aging, and can cause neurodegenerative problems such as Alzheimer's. Copper pots are also problematic. Acid foods in contact with the copper will leach harmful amounts of copper into the foods, causing numerous health problems as well as accelerating the aging process. Nonstick coatings on cookware are notoriously toxic, especially when heated to high temperatures, emitting fumes that have been linked to cancer and reproductive problems.

What's in Your Water?

According to a December 2009 analysis by the *New York Times,* more than 20 percent of the water treatment systems in the United States had violated the safety standards in the Safe Drinking Water Act during the prior five years. The *Times* found that about 50 million Americans had been drinking water with unsafe levels of toxins like arsenic and tetrachloroethylene, radioactive substances like uranium, prescription drugs, and dangerous sewage bacteria. Meanwhile, several studies in the *American Journal of Epidemiology* indicate that these chemicals cause harm at concentrations even lower than the existing standards. The *Times* said, "Studies indicate that drinking water contaminants are linked to millions of instances of illness within the United States each year."

Half of all groundwater wells contain pesticide and fertilizer residues. Phosphate fertilizers are a problem because they are often contaminated with cadmium. The cadmium gets into the groundwater and into the food, contributing to higher cancer rates. Phosphate fertilizers also accelerate the leaching of arsenic from soils into groundwater and plants. For example, phosphate-treated soil increases arsenic accumulation in wheat. Nitrates, primarily from nitrogen fertilizers, also end up in the drinking water. Nitrates in our environment and food have been linked to increased deaths from such diseases as Alzheimer's, diabetes, and Parkinson's.

A 2010 study by the Environmental Working Group found hexavalent chromium in the tap water of thirty-one out of thirty-five cities sampled. Hexavalent chromium is used in chrome plating and the manufacturing of plastics and dyes, and it has been linked to liver and kidney damage in animals, as well as to leukemia, stomach cancer, and other cancers.

Even if your water starts out pure, most tap water in the United States is treated with chlorine and fluoride and is unfit to drink. The fluoridation process introduces additional arsenic into the water. In 2001, the National Research Council warned, "Even very low concentrations of arsenic in drinking water appear to be associated with a higher incidence of cancer." These health-destroying toxins must be removed from your water.

Chlorine

Chlorine, added to kill bacteria, kills and injures your cells as well. If you drink, bathe, shower, or swim in chlorinated water, you are inhaling and absorbing chlorine into your body, damaging genes and cells. Exposure to vaporized chlorine in the shower is 100 times more damaging than drinking chlorinated water, because the inhaled gases go directly into the bloodstream. In fact, about two-thirds of our exposure to chlorine results from inhalation and skin absorption when showering. When chlorine reacts with organic compounds in the water, it forms highly toxic organochlorine compounds. Swimming pools and hot tubs can abound in these chemicals, which do not break down easily, and accumulate over time. The average American is accumulating more than 175 organochlorine compounds. Chlorine is not necessary to treat drinking water. There are safer alternatives. Use water filters to take out existing chlorine and organochlorine compounds.

Fluoride

Very simply, fluoride makes you old and sick; it is a general cellular poison, doing catastrophic biological damage to our population. Fluoride, added for supposed dental health benefits, is a waste product of the pollution-scrubbing devices of the phosphate fertilizer industry. In scientific circles, fluoridation has been known for decades as one of our greatest public health blunders. The evidence against fluoride is overwhelming, and it has been in the public domain for decades, despite attempts to obscure it. In the 1960s, researchers from Harvard University and the National Institutes of Health discovered that fluoride disrupted collagen synthesis. Since then, numerous studies all over the world have linked fluoride to both "old age" and "genetic" disorders, including wrinkled skin, arthritis, arteriosclerosis, brittle bones, heart disease, and cancer. Thyroid disease and neurodegenerative diseases, like Parkinson's and Alzheimer's, are both linked to fluoride and are now reaching epidemic proportions among baby boomers, who have been exposed to fluoride for most of their lives. Fluoride calcifies your pineal gland, which can lead to a number of health problems, from precocious puberty to cancer; both are burgeoning epidemics. In 2006, a committee of the National Research Council unanimously concluded that the EPA-approved levels of fluoride in the water were damaging to human health. Tragically, more than 60 percent of U.S. water supplies are currently fluoridated.

Fluoride Inhibits DNA Repairs

According to the National Academy of Sciences and the World Health Organization, at 1 part per million (ppm), the level commonly found in tap water, fluoride inhibits more than 100 enzymes in the body, including critical DNA repair enzymes. Numerous studies have shown that fluoride causes genetic damage. One reason why older people have more cancer is a decline in their ability to repair damaged DNA—1 ppm of fluoride can disrupt DNA repair enzymes by 50 percent.

The Fountain of Old Age

If there is such a thing as the "fountain of old age," your tap water is it. Fluoride in tap water blocks enzymes essential for producing intact collagen. The body uses collagen fibers to ensure structural integrity of tissues like skin, bone, muscle, ligaments, and tendons. It is collagen—both the soft, *unmineralized* type in our skin and joints, and the hard, *mineralized* type in our teeth and bones— that visually signals our age. Cumulative damage to collagen and collagen-producing cells leads to many conditions attributed to old age, such as arthritis, arteriosclerosis, brittle bones, and wrinkled skin. Consumption of fluoride produces these effects because it disrupts the normal mineralization of collagen, making you look and feel old.

Fluoride Teams Up with Other Toxic Chemicals

Heavy metals and other contaminants cause more harm in the presence of fluoride. For example, chloramines combined with fluoride in city water extract lead from old pipes. In addition to helping contaminate the water, the fluoride transports lead and other heavy metals to various areas of your body. It is known to increase lead accumulation in bones and teeth. It also helps toxic metals penetrate your brain—something they can't do on their own.

Are You Eating Your Fluoride?

According to Jeff Green, national director for Citizens for Safe Drinking Water, due to the widespread use of fluoride-based pesticides, nonorganic food accounts for as much as one-third of the average person's fluoride exposure. His group has discovered that nonorganic fresh produce, juices (particularly grape juice), lunchmeats, tea, and breakfast cereals are all contaminated with high doses of fluoride. Iceberg lettuce can contain up to 180 parts per million (ppm)—180 times the limit recommended in drinking water. Citrus fruits can contain up to 95 ppm of sodium aluminum fluoride. Raisins can have up to 55 ppm, and potatoes—up to 22 ppm on the outside and up to 2 ppm on the inside. Grapes can be a major source of fluoride because they're heavily sprayed with cryolite, a fluoride-based pesticide. This means anything made with nonorganic grapes is highly contaminated with fluoride. For example, juice drinks that people think of as healthy usually contain white grape juice, added as a sweetener. The average American is getting a daily dose of fluoride that far exceeds even the EPA's inadequate safety standards.

If It's So Bad, Why Do They Do It?

We've all heard that fluoride helps fight cavities. However, numerous studies show that fluoride does nothing to protect teeth. In fact, cities that fluoridate often have higher cavity rates. Fluoride damages your bones and teeth by binding to calcium and magnesium and creating deficiencies of these minerals. Robert Carton, PhD, a former risk assessment manager for the U.S. Environmental Protection Agency (EPA), said in an interview with the Canadian Broadcast Company's *Marketplace* on November 24, 1992, "Fluoridation is the greatest case of scientific fraud of this century." He added, "EPA has more than enough evidence to shut down fluoridation right now," and, "Fluoridation constitutes unlawful medical research. It is banned in most of Europe."

Most people are unaware that the FDA has never approved adding fluoride to drinking water. The FDA and the EPA have been dancing around this issue for decades in an attempt to avoid jurisdiction. Why don't they just ban the practice of fluoridating water? It's because of the legal liability. If we admit how toxic this stuff is, how many people have been given cancer, weak bones, and bad teeth, then the American Dental Association, dentists, water departments, toothpaste manufacturers, and the companies who sell these toxic chemicals would all be sued out of existence—it's almost unthinkable. So, the charade that fluoride is safe and beneficial continues.

It is essential to purify your drinking water. A high-quality reverse osmosis system removes fluoride, chlorine and chlorinated compounds, prescription drugs, arsenic, aluminum, and other toxins. Do not use fluoride toothpaste, and avoid processed foods. Buy organic as much as possible. Supplement with magnesium, calcium, and vitamin C. This helps bind the free fluoride ions and excrete them from your body more effectively.

Bottled Water

Is bottled water safe? If you can get it in glass bottles from a high-quality source, the answer is yes. The quality of bottled water varies widely, and many brands have been found no better, and in some cases worse, than ordinary tap water. In addition, toxins from the plastic bottles leach into the water. A 2009 study by the Environmental Working Group found an average of eight chemical contaminants in each of the ten popular bottled water brands sampled, some exceeding the legal limits for bottled water contaminants. Half the brands were contaminated with bacteria. Your safest bet is to use a high-quality, reverse osmosis water purification system at home, put this water in a glass bottle, and carry it with you.

The Air

It is estimated that 64,000 Americans die prematurely each year from heart and lung disease caused by particulate pollution. Inhaling small particles can disrupt the heart's beat-to-beat variations, increasing mortality risk from all causes. However, you don't have to live downwind of a power plant or drive behind a truck to be poisoned by air pollution. While you may think of your home as your castle, it may be more like a toxic waste dump. Toxicity from indoor air pollution affects most Americans, producing anxiety, depression, fatigue, headaches, poor concentration, and poor mental acuity, as well as bodily aches and pains. When people complain of these symptoms, however, their physicians almost never suggest indoor pollutants as a probable (or even possible) cause.

Airborne Particles

The average American breathes in two heaping tablespoons of airborne particles each day. The smallest of these are capable of lodging deep in the lungs, where they cause serious problems. In 2004, researchers reported in the journal *Science* that fine airborne particles can cause genetic mutations that are passed on to future generations. Most of these fine particles emanate from industrial plants, power plants, incinerators, and diesel-burning vehicles. In the MATES II report, a study of Los Angeles air concluded that 71 percent of the cancer risk from air contaminants came from diesel emissions. The harmful effects of air pollution may surface immediately, years later, or even in the next generation. Although specific health damage is often hard to pinpoint, even colds, flu, and asthma can result from impaired immunity caused by breathing polluted air.

To protect yourself from air pollution, you must begin with your personal environment. Carpets, mattresses, paints, cleaning supplies, gas appliances, fragrances, and deodorizers all introduce pollutants into your home and workplace. Install water and air filters in your home, especially if you live in a city or near a heavily traveled highway with diesel emissions. You can prevent genetic damage caused by fine particles by filtering your air with a HEPA (high-efficiency particulate air) filter.

Toxins in Your Home

Some of the most polluted air you can breathe is right in your own home. The EPA has found that most indoor air is two to five times more polluted than outdoor air, and it can easily be a hundred times more polluted due to the combined effects of multiple toxic sources concentrated in a confined space. Add to that the fact that most Americans spend 90 percent of their time indoors, and you are looking at a major aging and disease factor.

Virtually anything in your home can be a source of pollutants: building materials, furnishings, mattresses, gas appliances, furnaces, cleaning and personal care products, tobacco smoke, incense, deodorants, carpets, paint, copy machines, printers, electronic equipment, dry cleaning, newspapers, and magazines. Any smell that is not a natural smell is almost certainly toxic. Hot water in dishwashers, clothes washers, bathtubs, and showers vaporizes chlorine and other chemicals, as well as the bleaches or detergents being used. Good ventilation is essential, as is using a water filter for showering.

Obvious though it sounds, the most important thing you can do to keep your indoor air clean is to stop introducing pollutants in the first place. Before purchasing something, consider what it might add to your indoor pollution. If your new item has an odor, give it a chance to outgas before putting it in your living space. When you can, use heat or sunshine to expedite the outgassing process. Do not use products that have noticeable chemical odors, such as mothballs or air fresheners.

Building Materials

Building materials, such as plywood, particleboard, and paints, outgas formaldehyde, a common indoor pollutant and carcinogen. Formaldehyde causes serious damage to DNA, and the damage is cumulative as exposure continues. The industry will tell you that safer particleboards have been sold since the 1980s, but they outgas other toxic chemicals and are still not safe.

Carpets

Synthetic carpets outgas for decades. New carpets are especially toxic. As many as 200 toxic chemicals outgas from the fibers, dyes, adhesives, backing, fire retardants, fungicides, antistatic and stain-resistant treatments, and padding. Researchers at Anderson Laboratories, an independent materials testing laboratory, measured the effects of carpet toxicity on 110 families and found that 82 percent developed health problems within three months of installation, including irregular heartbeat, fatigue, rashes, memory loss, muscle pain, blurred vision, and tremors. A 1995 study in the *Journal of Nutritional and Environmental Medicine* found that mice exposed to new carpet fumes died in a matter of hours. Even carpets up to twelve years old caused neurological problems. Install only natural fiber carpets, tile, stone, bamboo, or hardwood floors with area rugs.

Appliances

Gas stoves, water heaters, furnaces, space heaters, and fireplaces release dangerous toxins into the indoor air. These include nitrogen dioxide, carbon monoxide, methane, and other gases, along with fine particles. Keep furnaces and gas water heaters outside the living space, preferably in a shed or unattached garage. If you have a gas water heater in your living space, consider switching to an electric water heater. Use gas stoves only with good ventilation; an electric stove is preferable. Use fireplaces sparingly, and never use artificial logs as they put out a heavy hydrocarbon load.

The Bathroom

Look in your bathrooms. Likely, there are enough toxins there to make anybody sick. In addition to the chlorinated water coming out of the tap, toilet bowl cleaners, hair spray, and deodorizers all release toxins into the air. Toilet deodorizers are made from paradichlorobenzene, the same toxic chemical found in mothballs. Replace all of these products with safer, simpler, yet effective items available in health food stores.

The Laundry Room

Do your eyes, nose, or throat feel irritated when you walk down the detergent aisle at the grocery store? Many people are sensitive to toxic fumes and residues from laundry detergents and fabric soft-eners. When washing your clothes, use environmentally friendly and unscented laundry products such as the Seventh Generation brand. Do not use scented fabric softeners; these products might make your clothes smell "clean and fresh," but that smell is toxic. Detergents, bleach, spot removers, and fabric softeners all contain toxic chemicals. Manufacturers have lulled us into complacency with the term "biodegradable," meaning that at some point the detergent will lose its foaming properties. This fact has little to do with the impact on your health or the environment. Purchase only unscented products. Synthetic detergents can be replaced with natural soap-based products, while chlorine bleach can be replaced with safer oxygen bleaches such as sodium percarbonate and hydrogen peroxide.

Furniture

Furniture is often made with synthetic materials (polyester, polyurethane, polystyrene, and polyvinyl chloride) that outgas toxins. Watch out for particleboard furniture covered with a wood or plastic veneer, which will outgas formaldehyde or other toxins. Alarmingly, most children's furniture is made with particleboard. Research shows that bringing particleboard furniture into an empty house can triple the formaldehyde levels in the air. Most homes today are made with particleboard, but mobile homes, where every-thing may be made from particleboard, are of special concern. Opt for solid wood or metal furniture, and look for used items to save money.

Clothing

Even the clothes you wear can be toxic. Have you ever noticed the chemical-laden atmosphere inside a clothing store? That odor is caused by toxins outgassing from synthetic fibers (nylon, polyester, acrylics, and spandex) in the clothes. Often clothes are treated with dyes, formaldehyde finishes (permanent press), and mothproofing pesticides. New or freshly dry-cleaned clothes bring toxins close to your body and into your household. Wash new clothes before you wear them and always air out your clothes after they've been dry-cleaned before you put them in your closet. For daily wear, buy clothes made of natural fibers—cotton, wool, linen, and silk. Hang cedar blocks in your closets as an alternative to mothballs.

Prescription Drugs

A major category of avoidable toxins is prescription drugs. When we finally get sick from our poor nutrition and toxic overload, we go to conventional physicians who unwittingly make us even sicker by increasing our toxic load with drugs. *Prescription drugs are so toxic that properly prescribed drugs are the third-leading cause of death in America.* If we outlawed prescription drugs, we could save hundreds of thousands of lives each year while also increasing our quality of life. Health would improve, and our health care costs would go down by hundreds of billions of dollars.

Drugs create completely new health problems, even though many are little better than placebos at controlling disease. Dr. Mehmet Oz, a professor of surgery at Columbia University and author of *YOU: The Owner's Manual,* had this to say: "For every dollar we spend on prescription drugs, we spend a dollar to fix a complication." The top-selling drug in the world is a cholesterol-lowering drug. Yet, a 1996 study in the *Journal of the American Medical Association* determined that "All members of the two most popular classes of lipid-lowering drugs (the fibrates and the statins) cause cancer in rodents, in some cases at levels of animal exposure close to those prescribed to humans."

Since the year 2000, sales of prescription drugs have more than tripled. Americans represent 4 percent of the world's population, yet they take 50 percent of all the prescription drugs produced in the world. Half of all Americans now take at least one prescription drug. One out of four children takes at least one prescription drug. Many of our elderly take a dozen or more drugs per day. It's no wonder they are losing their minds, unstable on their feet, and feeling fatigued, with their health spiraling downward. Alarming amounts of prescription drugs are now showing up in our water supply, poisoning fish, animals, and humans.

Because so many of us have taken antibiotics, which destroy the normal gut bacteria and allow yeast and fungi to grow, yeast infections are now a major source of toxicity. Yeast destroys enzymes needed for cell energy and releases DNA-damaging free radicals, causing fatigue and other symptoms. To eliminate yeast, drop sugar and grains from your diet, follow the suggestions in the chapters on nutrition (Chapters 3 and 4), and take high-quality supplements.

By the time you are on more than a couple of prescription drugs, every cell in your body is being poisoned, and no one in the world knows what is going on—you are in biochemical chaos. When your body is in chaos, this is disease. The healthiest person alive will get sick if they take prescription drugs. So how can a sick person expect to get well? Both prescription and over-the-counter drugs are unnecessary. There are very few instances where there is not a safer and more effective alternative to a drug. Our physicians have been taught that drugs are the answer to disease. In reality, drugs don't provide answers—they create problems.

Personal Care Products

Almost all personal care products such as toothpaste, soaps, shaving cream, aftershave, nail polish, deodorants, skin lotions, hair sprays, hair dyes, fragrances, shampoos, and conditioners contain toxic chemicals that add to your toxic overload and stress your immune system. At least one-third of the chemicals used in these products have already been identified as causing serious health problems. Most people don't even conceive that products as common as toothpaste or shampoo are significant sources of dangerous toxins that are making them sick and old. Seek out and use only safe personal care products.

Surprisingly, *putting chemicals in your mouth or on your skin can be 100 times more toxic than ingesting them.* Toxins you swallow are subjected to enzymes in your stomach and then pass through the liver, where they are broken down before they reach the rest of your body. When toxins are absorbed through the mucous membranes in the mouth or through the skin, they can directly enter the bloodstream and your tissues. Be especially cautious when choosing your mouthwash, toothpaste, shampoo, and skin lotions.

Most are highly toxic and cause serious damage as chemicals bioaccumulate in your cells and tissues with daily use.

Most skin creams contain a mixture of toxic chemicals including
mineral oil, paraffin, and petrolatum. These petroleum products are
suspected carcinogens and hormone disruptors. Parabens are the
usual preservatives in these products, and they too have hormone-
disrupting qualities. Sodium lauryl or laureth sulfate are included in
more than 90 percent of personal care products. They break down
the skin's moisture barrier, allowing other chemicals to penetrate
the skin, and they combine with other chemicals, forming powerful
toxins. Acrylamide is found in many hand and face creams, and is
known to react with DNA, potentially leading to DNA mutations.
Dioxane is a powerful toxin found as a contaminant in ingredients
such as PEG (polyethylene glycol), polysorbates, laureth, and eth-
oxylated alcohols. Other common toxic ingredients include phenol
carbolic acid and propylene glycol. Suntan lotions contain at least
half a dozen chemicals that have been found to be carcinogens or
endocrine disruptors.

To get an idea of how toxic your toothpaste is, read the warning label on the box. It most likely says something like, "Keep out
of reach of children under six years of age. If you accidentally
swallow more than used for brushing, seek professional help or
contact a poison control center immediately." There is a reason for
this warning. One tube is sufficient to kill a small child! Conventional toothpaste is a deadly mixture of numerous toxins: fluoride;
artificial colors, flavors, and sweeteners; synthetic detergents like
sodium lauryl sulfate (SLS); and others. All of these pass through

the mucous membranes and bioaccumulate in the body, leading to toxic overload, disease, and accelerated aging.

Shampoo is another toxin-loaded product that many use daily. Shampoos also usually contain SLS, which disrupts the nervous system, hormone system, and normal cell chemistry. In addition, SLS is frequently contaminated with 1,4-dioxane, which is toxic to the liver, kidneys, and brain. Dioxane has even been found in baby shampoo. Shampoos also contain preservatives such as paraben compounds. The EPA has linked parabens to hormonal, neurological, metabolic, and developmental disorders, and to cancer. Researchers have found parabens in every sample of breast cancer tissue. Propylene glycol is another chemical found in numerous shampoo and skincare products. It is a skin irritant and is known to cause liver and kidney damage. Shampoos also contain a variety of artificial colors and other toxic and carcinogenic chemicals. In a June 29, 2010, report titled *Food Dyes: The Rainbow of Risks,* the Center for Science in the Public Interest stated: "The three most widely used dyes, Red 40, Yellow 5, and Yellow 6, are contaminated with known carcinogens. . . . Another dye, Red 3, has been acknowledged for years by the Food and Drug Administration to be a carcinogen, yet is still in the food supply."

A 2007 study in the *International Journal of Cancer* revealed that monthly use of permanent hair dye doubled the risk of bladder cancer when used for twelve months. The risk tripled after fifteen years of use. Temporary or semipermanent dyes did not have the same risks, according to the researchers.

For many people, wearing perfume, cologne, or other artificial fragrances is as natural as wearing clothes. Yet even high-end perfumes are made with cocktails of dangerous and untested chemicals. According to the Environmental Working Group, most perfumes contain an average of ten known allergens, which can trigger reactions from asthma and headaches to contact dermatitis, and an average of four known endocrine disruptors that are linked to reproductive defects in men, and more recently, hyperactivity in children.

Most household cleaning products are made with toxic fragrances. The industry uses more than 5,000 different chemicals to make synthetic fragrances. Among them are endocrine disrupting chemicals like phthalates and toxic solvents like xylene and toluene. Toluene is found in most synthetic fragrances, and chronic exposure can cause anemia, low blood cell count, liver or kidney damage, and damage to a fetus. These ingredients are not regulated, and they do not need to be listed on the label. If you wish to use a fragrance, use a natural essential oil. These are derived from herbs and flowers and are available at health food and specialty stores.

Always read the ingredients of any personal care product you use and avoid the ones containing the known toxins I've described above. Fortunately, there are safe personal care products available at health food stores and other sources (see Appendix C). Choosing them will lower your toxic load, lessen the burden on your immune system, and help you stay healthy and biologically young.

Staying Safe on the Go

Commuting and traveling have become a big part of our lives and a big source of environmental toxins. As with everything, taking simple commonsense precautions will go a long way toward protecting your health.

Toxins in Your Car

New cars are particularly toxic. Plastics, adhesives, and seating materials pollute the interior air of the car with known endocrine disruptors and carcinogens. One class of these chemicals, phthalates, disrupts normal hormone function by mimicking estrogen. Phthalates are also found in plastic bottles, food packaging, hoses, shower curtains, vinyl wall coverings, toys, cosmetics, hair conditioners, and fragrances. During the first few months, try to leave a new car parked in the hot sun with the windows up to bake out the toxins. Air it out regularly, especially before you drive it, and keep it well ventilated while driving. Attached garages are another problem. Exhaust fumes and hydrocarbon vapors coming from a hot engine can enter the living space. Whenever possible, leave the garage door open to ventilate that space, especially after a long trip when the engine and oil are hot.

Hotels

Hotel rooms are heavily sprayed with pesticides. Nowadays, when so many people have chemical sensitivities, good hotels are starting to offer chemical-free rooms. Because hotel carpets, furniture, and mattresses are all relatively new, the toxic load in a typical room is enormous. It wouldn't be so bad if one could simply air the room. Unfortunately, most hotels now seal their windows. When making hotel reservations, remember to request a nonsmoking room, and always bring your own nontoxic soap and shampoo.

What to Eat When You Travel

It is a challenge to avoid toxic foods when traveling. Make the best choices you can under the circumstances. When I travel, I often eat fresh fruit for breakfast and salads for other meals.

Support Detoxification

To reduce our toxic load, first we have to learn where toxins come from and avoid them. Supporting the body's detoxification system is next. External pollutants from food, air, and water are only part of our toxic load. The rest comes from our own cells, which generate a huge amount of toxins every day as waste products of normal metabolism. Our bodies are built to safely dispose of these chemicals through exquisitely designed detoxification systems. Unfortunately, we are overloading these systems. Some of the external toxins we are exposed to disable them, and our diets fail to supply sufficient nutrients to keep the detoxification systems running.

How the Body Detoxifies Itself

The liver is your major detoxification organ. At any given time, about 25 percent of all the blood in your body is in your liver to be detoxified. This happens in two phases. In Phase 1, the liver produces enzymes that oxidize harmful toxins such as prescription drugs, alcohol, pesticides, and herbicides. This process creates harmful free radicals that must be neutralized with dietary antioxidants. In Phase 2, more enzymes are used to combine these oxidized chemicals with other molecules, so that they can be harmlessly excreted in the bile or urine. In both phases, the raw materials needed to produce enzymes, antioxidants, and other chemicals involved in the process come from the food we eat. When our diets consistently supply the correct nutrients, these elegant systems do a fabulous job. But that's not what usually happens.

How to Eat for Detoxification

Support your liver's Phase 1 detoxification process with antioxidant nutrients. Supplement with vitamins A, C, and E, along with CoQ_{10}, carotenoids, bioflavonoids, selenium, manganese, copper, and zinc. Some of these nutrients neutralize free radicals directly; others activate enzymes that neutralize them. Red, yellow, and green vegetables are loaded with these antioxidant nutrients.

Support Phase 2 detoxification with cruciferous vegetables, such as cabbage, broccoli, cauliflower, green onions, kale, and brussels sprouts. Many people know that broccoli is "good for them," because it is rich in vitamins A, C, and E, the big free radical scavengers. However, it is the sulfur compounds in broccoli and similar vegetables that signal human genes to express certain enzymes and activate detoxification. I recommend that you juice vegetables every day to get even more of the precious nutrients.

Remove Stored Toxins

As we grow older, our toxic load reaches disease-causing levels. Limiting our exposure to new toxins and supporting liver detoxification help to slow down the rate at which we accumulate new toxins. However, to reduce our overall toxic burden, we must actively purge stored toxins. Let's have a look at some of the things you can do to that end.

Saunas

Hyperthermic (sweat) treatments have been in use for millennia. The ancient Egyptians, Greeks, and Romans all used them, as did the cultures in the East. Native Americans used sweat lodges to treat diseases. The power of hyperthermic treatments lies in their ability to gently and effectively detoxify the body. The skin is the body's largest organ and an important part of the body's detoxification system. Saunas melt the fat layer in the skin, allowing the oil to ooze out of the oil glands along with its cargo of accumulated fat-soluble toxins, like pesticides and PCBs. In addition, sweat carries out water-soluble toxins, including heavy metals like lead and mercury. Over time, it is possible to reduce one's toxic load substantially, and then keep it low.

A regular dry sauna has become a necessity for achieving and maintaining health. Steam saunas and normal sweating will not do the job. By helping to remove toxins that interfere with cellular energy production, dry saunas support energy production and good health. Saunas are available at gyms and health clubs. If you use one of these commercial saunas, lie prone on the lowest bench. This will expose your body to a manageable temperature, allowing you to spend more time. A far-infrared sauna is the most effective way to remove stored toxins, but conventional saunas also work. The air temperature in an infrared sauna is lower, making it more pleasant than conventional saunas. I take a sauna for ninety minutes twice a week. If you have not used a sauna before, start by going in for a few minutes at a time and gradually work your way up. If you ever feel faint, dizzy, or sick, get out. After completing the sauna, immediately wash off with a good castile soap to get rid of the toxins before they reabsorb into the skin. It is important to keep hydrated when using a sauna. Drink pure water before, during, and after. Excessive water loss can disturb normal heart rhythms and cause dizziness, nausea, and fatigue.

Fasting

Fasting is the complete abstinence from all food except pure water, in a restful environment. Juice fasting, a popular variation, is abstinence from all food and drink except water and fresh vegetable juices. Fasting promotes detoxification. People have been fasting for thousands of years, both for spiritual and health purposes. It is an integral part of many religions, including Islam, Judaism, and Christianity. As far back as 400 BC, Hippocrates prescribed total abstinence from food while a disease was on the increase and a spare diet thereafter. Ancient priests provided sanctuaries for people to fast. Animals fast when they are sick or injured, and when we are sick, our hunger diminishes.

The body normally eliminates toxins through the colon, liver, kidneys, lungs, lymph nodes, and skin. During a fast, the body turns to its fat reserves for energy. When the fat is metabolized to make energy, it releases its stored toxins, which are then eliminated via the normal detoxification pathways. Fasting also triggers the healing process. The body uses lots of energy to digest food. When fasting, energy is diverted away from the digestive system and toward body metabolism and the immune system. The body searches for dead cells, damaged tissues, fatty deposits, tumors, and abscesses, and it takes them apart, burning them for fuel or expelling them as waste. During fasting, the body also rebuilds damaged tissues. Fasting allows the digestive system to repair itself, restoring good digestion and elimination.

A simple water fast works well for many people. Drink at least two liters per day of pure water to help flush toxins out of your system. Avoid water straight from the faucet. Distilled water from a pure, natural source or reverse osmosis water is best. Stir buffered vitamin C powder into water throughout the day for extra antioxidant power to protect against free radicals while helping the body to detoxify. Organic lemon juice in pure water is also helpful for cleansing, as lemon is especially supportive to the liver. If you wish to make fasting a habit, an excellent book is *Toxic Relief* by Don Colbert, MD.

If you have responsibilities to maintain during your fast, you may find you have a little more energy with a juice fast. Consume a few eight-ounce glasses of fresh, homemade vegetable juice (not store-bought processed juice) throughout the day. The vegetable juice also provides antioxidant protection from the toxins being released into your system as your body detoxifies.

Fasting is not for everyone. Some individuals do not fast well due to blood sugar issues. Cancer of the liver is another instance where fasting is contraindicated. However, in some situations, fasting is the only known solution. Fasting helps to dissolve tumors, and many patients have overcome cancer with fasting. It has also been beneficial for many other health problems, including addictions, arthritis, asthma, chronic fatigue, colitis, Crohn's disease, hypertension, lupus, and even some mental illness. To cure a severe disease, it is usually necessary to continue through a series of fasts.

Fasting is the one practice that has been proven to extend life. Dr. Roy Walford, author of *The Anti-Aging Plan*, showed that mice that fasted two days a week doubled their life span and were healthier. Making a habit of fasting one day a week is not difficult, and by doing so, your body gets fifty-two days a year to rest and detoxify. Some people prefer to fast three or four days in a row each month. Unless you have problems with blood sugar, this is safe and beneficial. If you are not sure about blood sugar problems, check with your doctor. I normally fast one day per week, and once a year, I fast for seven to ten days; I feel fantastic afterward. In fact, it was a ten-day fast that helped me recover from liver failure caused by a toxic prescription drug. Longer fasts are preferable to short ones, because once the body is in the fasting state, systemic cleansing is able to reach into the harder-to-get-at body tissues. Many recoveries from serious illnesses have taken place with longer fasts.

As your body eliminates more and more toxins, you will notice increased energy, better health, and sharper mental functioning.

Regular fasting is one habit that will reward you with innumerable benefits, including healthy weight, a younger body, and a longer life.

Enemas

   Like fasting and saunas, enemas have been in use since the dawn of civilization. In ancient Egypt, the enema was deemed so essential that every pharaoh had a special physician appointed as "Guardian of the Anus." Enemas detoxify the body by flushing the large intestine. They are also known today as colonic hydrotherapy or colonics.

   The colon completes the process of digestion and elimination. Enzyme-deficient processed foods, excess proteins, refined sugars, improper food combining, lack of nutrients and probiotic bacteria, sedentary lifestyles, and stress—all combine to hinder our digestion and leave large amounts of partially digested food particles in the colon. As a result, the colon becomes sluggish. The healthy transit time of food through our body is less than twenty-four hours. For many people today, this time is up to seventy hours. During this time, the contents of your large intestine breed unhealthy bacteria and release toxins that get reabsorbed into the bloodstream. Cleansing the colon helps detoxify and rejuvenate the whole body. It is especially recommended at the end of a prolonged fast, as the body rids itself of the stored toxins. Colonics are typically performed by licensed health practitioners at naturopathic clinics and other wellness centers.

Coffee Enemas

Another effective approach to detoxification is coffee enemas—not recommended if you are allergic to coffee. Coffee enemas work well in conjunction with vegetable juicing to heal the body, particularly of cancer. They were already an established part of medical practice when the famous cancer pioneer Dr. Max Gerson introduced them into cancer therapy in the 1930s. Coffee enemas stimulate liver enzymes that are vital for detoxification and help break down carcinogenic compounds. Coffee contains substances called choleretics, which help dilate and open up the bile ducts to allow drainage of toxins from the liver. There is excellent information on how to do coffee enemas in print and on the Internet. Another option to help reduce inflammation in the body is vitamin C enemas using buffered vitamin C.

Vitamin C Flush

A vitamin C flush is like an internal enema that benefits the entire digestive system and the body as a whole. It helps to eliminate toxins, but also to reduce inflammation and rebuild healthy gut tissue. Take vitamin C to bowel tolerance; that is, until you reach a watery stool or an enema-like evacuation of liquid from the rectum. It is best to start first thing in the morning on an empty stomach. Allow yourself the rest of the day to finish the flush. Most people saturate their ascorbate need within a few hours. Occasionally, the need is much greater, and it may take most of the day to complete the flush.

Dissolve the fully reduced, mineral-buffered L-ascorbate powder in half a glass of water. (Count and record each dosage.) Wait for the fizz to settle, and then drink. The amount of L-ascorbate you need depends on how quickly your body uses it up. Below are a few suggestions:

A healthy person begins with a level half teaspoon dissolved in water or diluted juice every fifteen minutes.

A moderately healthy person begins with one teaspoon every fifteen minutes.

A person in ill health begins with two teaspoons every fifteen minutes.

If after four doses there is no gurgling or rumbling in the gut, double the initial dosage and continue every fifteen minutes.

Do not stop at loose stool. Continue with these instructions until a quart or so of liquid is expelled from the rectum. You want to energize the body to flush out toxins and reduce the risk that they may recirculate and cause problems. After the flush, stop consuming the buffered ascorbate for the day. However, if your flush dosage is more than fifty grams of vitamin C, you should consume a dosage of vitamin C of at least 10 percent of that during the remainder of the day.

Caution: It is critical that the vitamin C used is very pure and contains a proper balance of the major essential buffering minerals: potassium, magnesium, calcium, and zinc. The label should read: 100 percent L-ascorbate, fully reduced, corn-free, buffered mineral ascorbate.

The Bad and the Good

The bad news is we live in a toxic world and most of us are in toxic overload. Toxins make us sick and accelerate the aging process. After reading this chapter, you may feel discouraged because toxins are everywhere and avoiding them is impossible. While toxins are everywhere in our environment, there is good news. There is much you can do to lessen the impact of our toxic world. With even just a few good choices, you can reduce your toxic load substantially and support your body's detoxification processes so that it can handle the problem.

Use the information in this chapter to identify where most of your toxic exposures are coming from. Work to eliminate, or at least reduce, those exposures. Improve your diet and take high-quality supplements to support your detoxification pathways. Actively work to reduce your existing toxic burden with frequent saunas. Toxins damage tissue and interfere with the repair process, so if you learn to move yourself in the right direction on the Toxin Pathway, it will help limit the damage and switch your body back into the repair mode. When your cells are actively repairing themselves, you will be reducing your biological age and keeping yourself healthy and young. Think of the 100-year-old car that still looks and runs like new because it has been well maintained—you can do this, too.

The Bottom Line ━━━━━━━━━━━━━━━━━━━━━━━━━

✓ A toxin is any substance that causes a cell to malfunction. Toxicity is one of the two causes of all disease. A major reason that we get sicker as we age is that we become progressively more toxic.

✓ Although our bodies are designed to eliminate toxins, we live in a time of unprecedented toxic exposures from man-made chemicals. This deluge of toxins has exceeded our capacity to detoxify them. As a result, virtually every American is in toxic overload, storing and accumulating toxins in our body tissues that we have been unable to eliminate. These toxins age us and make us sick.

✓ But the situation is far from hopeless if we're willing to be proactive. We can reduce at least 80 percent of our toxic load by making good choices about those aspects of our environment that are under our control, especially in our home environment. This is sufficient to keep us healthy and biologically young.

✓ There are three ways to reduce your toxic load: (1) reduce the number of toxins coming in; (2) use good nutrition to support your body's detoxification pathways; (3) use specific therapies to remove stored toxins.

✓ To reduce the number of toxins coming in, educate yourself using the information in this chapter. Virtually anything in your personal environment is a possible source of toxicity: food and food packaging, cookware, water, building materials and furnishings, appliances, personal care products, cleaning products, clothing, etc. When considering a new purchase, evaluate its possible toxic impact. Gradually replace toxic products with nontoxic ones. Also make use of high-quality air and water purifiers.

✓ To support your body's detoxification pathways, eat ten to twelve servings of fruits and vegetables daily, especially vegetables that are red, yellow and green, and the cruciferous vegetables (like broccoli, cauliflower, brussels sprouts, cabbage, etc.). Juice vegetables to extract extra nutrients. Also increase antioxidant support with supplements like vitamins A, C, and E, CoQ_{10}, carotenoids, bioflavonoids, and the minerals selenium, manganese, copper, and zinc.

✓ To remove stored toxins, employ the following therapies: regular saunas, fasting, enemas, and the vitamin C flush.

CHAPTER 6

The Mental Pathway

*This is the great error of our day in the
treatment of the human body, that the physicians
separate the soul from the body.*

—Plato, *Charmides*

*People are just as happy as they
make up their minds to be.*

—Abraham Lincoln

W HY LIVE LONG IF YOU ARE GOING TO BE UNHAPPY? In fact, chances are you won't. A direct link between happiness and health is hardwired into your body. Positive thoughts of love, joy, compassion, and gratitude improve the immune system and support health, while anger, apathy, gloom, and resentment age you prematurely and ruin your health. In fact, the power of the mind to heal and rejuvenate, or to make you old and sick, is almost limitless. Good news or bad news? That all depends on your point of view.

Do you let worry and other toxic thoughts and emotions take over your mind? Do you give your power away to circumstances beyond your control? Or do you powerfully create mental states consistent with your long-term goals of being healthy and biologically young, regardless of your circumstances? In this chapter, I will show you how to use the mind as a pathway to staying youthful and strong, no matter what your age. Then I urge you to take action and experience for yourself the difference you can make by changing the way you think.

My Own Story:
"Every Day in Every Way I Get Stronger. . . ."

When I was dying of liver failure along with three auto-immune syndromes, chemical sensitivity, chronic fatigue, seizures, and a host of other problems, it occurred to me that, for survival, I needed to employ my mind as well as my body. I began to repeat to myself, again and again: *Every day in every way I get stronger and stronger and better and better.* At first, as I said this to myself, my mind would fight back, saying something like: *Wow, are you a liar! You are feeling worse with each passing day.* I saw that my own thinking was negating my efforts to stay positive and strong. I began to reply to my mind's objections by saying: *I know I feel worse today, but I am giving you an instruction.*

Once I became comfortable giving my body instructions, my own objections began to disappear and my body began to respond. I would say my affirmation, sometimes out loud, with passion and expectancy, many times daily, until I could feel strength coming into my body as I said the words. After a few weeks, my subconscious mind started acting on the instructions and the intent of my conscious mind. One day, after saying the affirmation, I felt the best that I had felt since I had fallen ill. The feeling lasted only minutes, but it proved that it was possible to feel better and that I was on the right path. Soon, the feelings of strength came more often and lasted longer. My badly damaged immune system was responding!

It was through this deeply personal experience that I began to understand that health and disease could be the reactions of the subconscious to the thoughts of the conscious mind. The subconscious takes orders from the conscious and puts them into action. Minds do what they are programmed to do. The trouble is that much of that programming is unintended. I began to realize my power to influence my health by choosing the daily thoughts I was putting into my head. By focusing on aging and disease, as I was originally programmed to do, I created more aging and more disease. When I focused the mind on what little strength I had left, even as I was on the brink of death, I threw the awesome powers of the mind on the side of recovery. The mind is always working, so why not make it work *for* rather than against you?

Aging Starts in the Mind

After my recovery, I began to study the biological connection between the mind and the immune system, our first line of defense against aging and disease. What I learned set me free from the conventional view that my chronological age defined my state of health and well-being. I discovered that it was not my age, but rather my mental attitudes toward aging and the other pressures of daily living that mattered most. The mind controls everything in the body, including aging. The way we perceive and react shows up on the cellular level. A 2002 study in the *Journal of Personality and Social Psychology* found that how you perceive aging affects how long you live. Those with more positive perceptions of their own aging lived an average of seven years longer. *That makes positive attitude more effective in extending life than low blood pressure, low cholesterol, healthy weight, or regular exercise.* The fountain of youth is right in your own mind!

The mind controls the body, and you control the mind. My journey on the path of healthy aging began with a thought that I chose to put into my head. That thought was to choose health and to create a lifestyle consistent with health. Now that I had experienced firsthand the power of the mind in creating health, I was determined to choose my thoughts just as carefully as I chose my food and my toothpaste. If you want to stay biologically young, you need to do the same thing. Here's why.

Every Thought Has a Biological Consequence

Happy people live longer. A 2011 study in *Biological Psychiatry* found that aging successfully is linked with a choice to live a happy, productive life. Approaching life's experiences with a positive attitude provides emotional and physical resilience throughout life, as well as longer life. The lesson to be learned is to use your mind to focus on the positive. A change in your thinking or beliefs can actually change how your genes express—same genes, different results.

Every thought and emotion triggers the release of chemical messengers throughout the body. Your emotional well-being and your physical health, to a large degree, depend on these chemical messengers. By producing a large variety of biologically active chemicals, every thought has a physical consequence. Your brain is the master of your nervous system, and your nervous system controls all the other systems in your body. Constantly repeating actions, thoughts, and words directly affects how our cells operate, influencing our health and the aging process for better or for worse. The CDC has stated that 85 percent of all diseases have an emotional component, and this estimate is most likely conservative.

Lack of purpose, low self-esteem, helplessness, hopelessness, anxiety, loneliness, depression, extreme mental or physical stress, or stressful life events, such as the loss of a loved one, have all been proven to be immune-suppressing. The membranes surrounding the cells of our immune system contain receptors for various neurochemicals produced in the brain, so the brain is directly communicating with immune cells. When we are happy, the brain produces a type of neurochemical that causes the immune system to strengthen and build. When we are stressed or depressed, the brain produces another type of neurochemical that effectively shuts down the immune system. Modern research has shown that negative thinking depresses the activity of immune system cells, natural killer (NK) cells, and T- and B-lymphocytes. When a person gives up and feels that life is no longer worth living, the immune system gives up as well.

Everyday emotional stress depletes the body of vital nutrients and produces toxic chemicals, creating deficiency and toxicity, the two causes of premature aging and disease. Stress, through a number of biochemical mechanisms, dramatically curtails the ability of cells to produce energy, and less energy reduces the body's ability to detoxify and provide for its normal functions. Yet many people needlessly stress themselves daily about things over which they have absolutely no control. Why do this? All you achieve is massive harm—to yourself! It's not worth the price.

What Is Stress?

In the mid-1970s, Hans Selye, MD, was the first to demonstrate that animals subjected to mental stress experienced depressed immunity, elevated blood pressure, elevated triglycerides, and stomach ulcers. Since then, thousands of human studies have shown a direct link between stress and disease. But what exactly is stress? We frequently equate mental stress with outward struggles: money, jobs, relationships, health, loss of loved ones, and so on. Most often, however, health-damaging, long-term stress comes from self-defeating beliefs and negative attitudes that we bring from our past. When we allow past fears and disappointments to rule our emotions and shape the way we experience the present, we end up living and reliving the same emotional trauma without ever realizing it.

Sally's Story: Living in the Past

Sally was in her mid-fifties when she came to me for help. Her health had been rapidly declining for some time. Now, on top of her numerous health problems, she had been diagnosed with cancer. When I spoke with her, I found out that twenty years prior she had gone through a nasty divorce. Then, every day since then, she had relived the stress of that divorce—running the same movie over and over in her mind. Painful memories and feelings became such a familiar part of her life that Sally didn't relate to them as stress. If anyone had asked Sally at that time whether she had been under a lot of stress, she would have wholeheartedly denied it. Yet her body was receiving a massive dose of stress hormones, day after day, until it destroyed her health and gave her cancer. Through psychotherapy, Sally was able to learn how to release her painful memories and think positive thoughts. In addition, she changed her diet and detoxified her body. Through these, Sally was able to cure her cancer.

How Stress Hormones Make You Old

In response to stress, your body releases a flood of hormones into your bloodstream. Hormones are part of your body's communication system. They deliver messages to cells and genes, acting as genetic switches turning genes on or off, and directly influencing important cellular processes, including cell repairs. Stress causes the release of growth-promoting hormones that help to switch on cancer. Stress hormones make blood platelets sticky, causing them to form clots, contributing to strokes and heart attacks. Stress hormones also activate an inflammatory response, which has been implicated in aging and degenerative diseases. At the same time, vital functions such as digestion, tissue repair, and immune response are put on hold and slowed down.

Subjecting yourself to persistently high stress is not a good idea. The constant onslaught of stress hormones will cause your cells to malfunction. According to 1996 data published by the CDC, stress-related problems account for up to 90 percent of the doctor visits in the United States. There is also direct scientific evidence that stress makes you old. In a study published in the 2013 *Proceedings of the National Academy of Sciences,* researchers found that caring for a child with a serious illness shortened the telomeres in the mother's cells, a result consistent with accelerated aging. Moreover, the study found the same result in mothers of healthy kids who reported burnout levels of stress. They had lost the telomere length equivalent to ten years of aging! Another study looked at people caring for Alzheimer's patients—an emotionally and physically stressful task, often requiring 100 or more hours per week. The researchers measured several markers of biological age among this group, including lymphocytes (part of the immune system), cytokines (a marker of inflammation), and telomere length. They found that the caregivers' biological age was up to *twenty years* older than their chronological age.

Norepinephrine, a hormone produced during periods of stress, increases the heart rate, blood pressure, and muscle tension. Norepinephrine also increases the growth rate of cancers by stimulating tumor cells to produce two collagen-dissolving enzymes that break down the tissue around the tumor cells. This allows cancer cells to move more easily into your bloodstream. Once in the bloodstream, these cells travel to other organs and tissues, forming new tumors.

Cortisol is secreted by the adrenal gland in response to stress. This hormone redirects energy (glucose) to parts of the body directly involved in fight-or-flight—the brain and major muscles. Cortisol suppresses the body's immune system. It has also been linked to increasing forgetfulness as we age. A 2011 study by the University of Edinburgh, in the *Journal of Neuroscience*, found that, while small amounts of cortisol improve memory, too much cortisol from chronic stress activates brain processes that lead to memory loss. Cortisol also causes inflammation and breaks down collagen, which leads to sagging skin and wrinkles.

Adrenaline is another hormone we produce more of when we are stressed. Adrenaline depresses immunity by decreasing available antibodies and reducing both the number and activity of lymphocytes. It decreases blood flow to the digestive tract, while pumping the blood out to the arms and legs. Unfortunately, any stress that we perceive in our mind will cause us to secrete adrenaline, whether we are in a combat zone, in rush-hour traffic, or thinking about a stressful event from the past.

The combined action of stress hormones is to redirect energy and nutrients toward muscles and major organs and away from organs and tissues not directly involved in the stress response, like skin and hair. Over time, elevated levels of stress hormones lead to overworking some parts of the body while starving others. Hypertension, fatigue, stiff muscles and joints, aches and pains, dry and wrinkled skin, and gray hair—practically all the signs of what we think of as normal aging—are linked to persistently high levels of stress.

Stress Less

People react to stress in different ways. Depending on how each chooses to respond, the same stressful event will make one person sick yet have no effect on another. Chronic stress releases a flood of tissue-damaging free radicals, creating chronic inflammation. Chronic inflammation damages tissue and causes aging; it is a major reason why older people become frail. To prevent accelerated aging, stress must be managed. We all live with stress. What matters is how you handle that stress. Depending on how you react, you can think your way into aging or you can think your way out of it. That California study of mothers caring for a chronically sick child found that the mothers who viewed their situation positively didn't suffer as much stress-related damage. These mothers often spent time learning about their child's condition and connecting with others in the same predicament or those willing to help. You see, it's all in how you look at it. When your outlook is stressing you and adding years to your biological age, it's time to change your outlook. It's that simple. Research confirms that a positive outlook on life and the support of friends help buffer a damaging stress response. In fact, the strength of friendships is an even stronger indicator of longevity than being married. Make and keep good friends.

Use Intention to Turn Your Mind into Your Ally

As a result of decades of research, we now know that cell chemistry can be directly influenced by human intention. This knowledge helps to explain the placebo effect, spontaneous remission, and the value of faith and prayer in human health. Thousands of years of human history tell us that the mind has a major impact on the body. There are even hundreds of research studies indicating that when conventional medicine's drugs and surgery work, it is because of the patient's belief in their efficacy. Belief is so powerful that it can even overcome the damage done by drugs and surgery and make you well. How much better it would be to harness that belief and skip the drugs and surgery altogether.

Our genes run the show, but the same genetic code produces different results based on the instructions we give to the genes. A strong and unambiguous intention to heal and stay well gives the genes the instructions to produce health-enhancing chemicals. Positive thoughts release "happy" brain chemicals, such as enkephalins and endorphins. Both these chemicals increase the production of immune T cells. But in addition to producing more

T cells, positive thoughts cause something magical to happen—the vigor with which the T cells attack the disease is also increased. Like nutrient-rich foods, positive thoughts increase immunity, protecting against aging and disease. Negative thoughts, similar to toxic overprocessed foods, do just the opposite!

Watch Your Thoughts

Make a habit of "eavesdropping" on your thoughts. Look for negative thoughts. For example, do you really think you are too old to change? Replace them with positive ones. You can change for the better at any time in your life. Take each negative thought and turn it around. It's amazing how much automatic negative thinking we do, but once you start paying attention and making different choices, you will do less and less of it.

Unchallenged negative thinking erodes self-confidence and undermines attempts to make things better. On the other hand, positive thinking creates new possibilities for happiness and health. There are good, scientifically sound reasons why people with positive outlooks live longer and healthier lives, while enjoying life far more than those with negative outlooks.

Choose Happiness

Many decades ago, I served a tour of duty in a U.S. Army combat infantry division. I knew at the outset that I would be separated from friends, family, and loved ones, and that there would be some unpleasant experiences. I knew I was going to live through these unpleasant experiences because I didn't have a choice. The only real choice was to be miserable or to be happy while experiencing them. I chose happy, and happily lived through some very miserable experiences. You can approach your life in the same way.

When life is filled with pain, sorrow, and disappointment, you can still choose to be happy regardless of the outward circumstances. Many autobiographies tell powerful stories about maintaining an unshakable optimism in the face of tremendous adversity. A positive outlook is often the secret behind surviving and beating the odds, be it a Nazi death camp or old age and disease. Think about and be grateful for the blessings you have. It's the choice that supports your immune system and your health. It's also more fun. Remember, happy comes from the inside. It's a big mistake to depend on things outside of us for our happiness.

Once you make up your mind to be happy, life gets better and everything becomes easier. Admittedly, no one is going to be happy all the time, but if you choose to be happy, most of the time, you will be. It will not only make you healthier, but will help you get through even the worst of times. Be a smile millionaire—the more you smile, laugh, and look on the bright side, the richer your life will be. Knowing you can choose to be happy is liberating. You don't have to feel bad because you're getting older, or because your life isn't going exactly as you planned. Once you make your mind up to be happy, you actually don't have to feel bad for any reason.

One of the greatest gifts you can give yourself is to choose happiness. Too often, we think that happiness is something that comes from outside us, but it really starts on the inside. There are people who have every advantage in life and are still not happy. Wealth, status, and material goods do not create happiness. It is a positive attitude that matters. Older people with positive attitudes have a 55 percent lower risk of death from all causes. Your attitude is something you choose, and the more you stay genuinely positive, the better your health outcome will be.

Serve a Purpose

One way to be happy is to have purpose in your life—pursuing what motivates and excites you. Think about what gives you the most satisfaction, and do something with it. Without purpose, life can be really dull, and your immune system will respond accordingly. We spend so much of our lives managing our fears, protecting ourselves from real or imaginary woes. Having a positive purpose can fundamentally shift your focus from things you do not want in your life to things you do want for yourself and others. How much more inspiring and uplifting!

Say It Out Loud

Simply stating your intentions makes a difference. Just as I did when I was hopelessly ill, many people have used affirmations to create breakthrough results in areas of life that matter to them. Keep your images and suggestions as positive, simple, clear, and concise as possible. Then repeat them as often as possible. Allow the subconscious to accept them as a "command." When the mind speaks, on some level the body listens.

Attention and Intention: Your Access to Power

It's hard to be happy when you feel powerless against your circumstances. The truth is that when it comes to your health, you are in the driver's seat. Two things are key to feeling empowered under any conditions: attention and intention. To make a difference in the physical world, including in your body, you have to pay attention to what it is you want to change and then form an intention of what you would like it to change into, even if the path is unclear.

Numerous scientific experiments have now proven what many people have preached for thousands of years—attention and intention can change your physical world. Change is best achieved when people enter into a calm, meditative state and then focus their attention and intention on what they want. In short, miracles can happen when people are in a calm mental and emotional state. Love, compassion, spiritual awareness, and all the life-affirming and positive emotions have extremely powerful implications for health and beyond. While these complex and intangible mental states are difficult to define, explain, or measure, they are perhaps the most "real" considerations in our lives. The will to live, choosing to be happy, and maintaining a state of inner peace and calm are keys to staying healthy and biologically young.

Is it realistic for an ordinary person to attain a mental and emotional state consistent with the highest potential for health and longevity? The answer is yes, and the method is various forms of spiritual practice. In this chapter, I will discuss two: meditation and prayer. Medical science has now confirmed what believers have known for millennia: prayer and meditation bring about measurable changes in health and biological age.

As you think about the power of your mind, consider what Deepak Chopra had to say in *Quantum Healing*: "Before this, science declared that we were physical machines that had somehow learned to think. Now it dawns that we are thoughts that have learned to make a physical machine."

Meditation

The meditative state is one in which normal thinking is suspended and you enter into the realm of pure awareness. If you haven't meditated in the past, it will take some practice to get rid of the mental chatter, quiet your mind, and focus on your true intentions—the rewards are worth the effort.

In 2009, a study in *NeuroImage* discovered that the brains of long-term meditators were physically different from those of nonmeditators. Brains normally shrink with age, and this may be responsible for many cognitive problems, but the brains of meditators have far less age-related shrinkage. Not only that, but follow-up research in 2011 in *NeuroImage* showed that the meditators had stronger connections between different parts of the brain. Even better, a 2011 study in *Psychiatry Research: Neuroimaging* found that a half-hour a day of mindful meditation (which focuses on nonjudgmental awareness of sensations, feelings, and state of mind) produced measurable changes in the parts of the brain associated with memory, sense of self, empathy, and stress in just eight weeks.

Meditation can even help with brain disease. A 2010 study in the *Journal of Alzheimer's Disease* demonstrated that meditation can lessen and possibly reverse the effects of Alzheimer's disease. Practicing meditation for only twelve minutes a day for eight weeks was shown to increase brain activity in areas important to memory, improved cognition, and well-being in patients with memory loss. Perhaps one reason for all these benefits is the telomere-repairing enzyme telomerase. Meditation activates this enzyme, which stimulates repairs, keeping your telomeres longer and you younger.

In Ayurvedic medicine, a deep level of relaxation is considered a precondition for healing. To restore health, the body must be brought back into balance, and meditative practice works to balance the body. Aging and disease happen when the body is out of balance. The body has many "natural rhythms," including something called heart-rate variability. Regular meditation helps to normalize these biological rhythms, bringing the body back into balance and good health. When the body's rhythms are rebalanced, fewer inflammatory chemicals are produced, more anti-inflammatory chemicals are produced, and NK cell activity is enhanced. Regular meditation is known to reduce stress, reduce inflammation, help regulate blood-sugar levels, and enhance immune function. Not surprisingly, the health literature contains many cases of people curing life-threatening illnesses through nothing more than diet and meditation. In truth, everyone should take time out to meditate every day.

Learning how to meditate is an investment in your future health, and there are many good books on how to do this. Don't be concerned that there are so many different meditating techniques. Choose one that works for you. If you develop the habit of meditating regularly week after week, you will develop an inner peace that is very beneficial to your health and longevity.

Aging is a multifaceted and complex process. Because of this, we must use every tool at our disposal to protect ourselves from unnecessary and premature aging. Your mind is one of the most powerful tools of all, and it doesn't cost anything to use it. *Put it to work and choose happy, loving thoughts and the belief that you will stay biologically young. Letting this seep into your subconscious through relaxed meditation can work miracles.*

Prayer

Dr. Larry Dossey, in his book *Healing Words*, describes the benefit of prayer as "one of the best kept secrets in medical science." Dr. Dossey defines prayerfulness as a feeling of love, compassion, and empathy toward another, and he explains that prayer is a powerful and legitimate (if often overlooked) method of healing. Now, medical research has shown that active faith really is good for you; it can make you healthier and happier, and it can motivate you to live longer as well. An analysis of more than 1,500 medical studies "indicates people who are more religious and pray more have better mental and physical health," says Dr. Harold G. Koenig, director of Duke University's Center for Spirituality, Theology, and Health. What's more, he says, "The benefits of devout religious practice, particularly involvement in a faith community and religious commitment, are that people cope better. In general, they cope with stress better, experience greater well-being, have more hope, are more optimistic, experience less depression [and] less anxiety, and commit suicide less often. They have stronger immune systems, lower blood pressure, and probably better cardiovascular functioning."

Study after study backs up the benefits of having faith, especially in prolonging life. According to a 2000 study in *Health Psychology*, there is a seven-year difference in life expectancy between those who never attend church and those who attend weekly. A study in the *American Journal of Public Health* followed nearly 2,000 older Californians for five years and found that those who attended religious services were 36 percent less likely to die during that period than those who didn't. A 2000 study of nearly 4,000 older adults in the *U.S. Journal of Gerontology* revealed that atheists had a significantly increased chance of dying earlier than the faithful. Crucially, religious people lived longer than atheists, even if they didn't go regularly to a place of worship. The American Society of Hypertension determined in 2006 that people who were involved in religious activities had significantly lower blood pressure than those who were not. Other studies revealed that believers recover from breast cancer quicker than nonbelievers, and have better outcomes from coronary disease and rheumatoid arthritis. An arthritis treatment center in Florida used prayer sessions to help alleviate pain. The patients who participated in the study showed "significant overall improvement" for up to one year later. In a study of nearly 92,000 people in Maryland, people who attended church once or more a week had 50 percent fewer deaths from coronary artery disease, 56 percent fewer deaths from emphysema, 74 percent fewer deaths from cirrhosis, and 53 percent fewer suicides.

Keep Your Brain Young

When used with attention and intention, the mind is the greatest healing tool of all. But in order to give the important matters in your life, like your health, your undivided attention and a clear intention, a healthy, active, and biologically young brain is a must. Science, which has long regarded the adult brain as static or declining, has recently discovered its plasticity—the ability of the brain to be readily shaped by experience. Research increasingly shows the adult human brain to be capable of forming new neural connections, even in the last decades of life, but it is up to us to help that happen.

Be a Lifetime Learner

Maintaining a youthful brain is a matter of "use it or lose it." Yes, brain function tends to peak by age thirty and then begin a slow decline. A 2012 study published in the *British Medical Journal* found measureable decline in brain function as early as age forty-five. But brain function can be improved at any age. Just as you need exercise to maintain a fit body, you need to challenge your brain with mental exercise. This becomes more important as you enter middle age and continues to be important for the remainder of life. Coping with new environments, learning and practicing a new skill, and challenging your higher cognitive powers by solving problems all strengthen existing neural connections and forge new ones.

In a 2012 interview by the Kavli Foundation, prominent brain researcher Dr. Michael Merzenich explained that age-related cognitive decline is caused by the way we use our brains. "When we're older," he said, "we spend most of the day operating automatically using skills and abilities that we developed in early life. . . . We avoid challenges, surprises and problems. . . . The average person can't describe the details of the street they live on. Because the brain hasn't been learning, its learning machinery is down regulated." He said numerous studies in both animals and humans have shown that it is possible to "sharply reverse all of the brain deficits linked to aging with training."

Live Mindfully

The trick is to get out of our ruts and approach life with a child's curiosity and openness to new experience. Mindfulness training, used in treating brain disorders and to reverse age-related cognitive decline, teaches us to "come to our senses," to hear, smell, taste, feel and really see the world around us as if for the first time—directly and free from judgments and other pre-conceived ideas. This exercises the way the brain takes in detailed information, and strengthens cognitive abilities that tend to decline with age like memory and information processing. Take a relaxed walk through your neighborhood just being present for what is here now. When you get home, close your eyes and recall your experience in as much sensory detail as you can. It is possible to "wake up" in any moment of your everyday life by simply shifting your attention from thinking to sensing.

Read

Reading helps you acquire new information, challenge old beliefs, and exercise your brain plasticity. Without curiosity and a desire to learn new things, your world begins to shrink and you begin shutting down. This is a primary cause of premature aging. Reading this book with its new facts and ideas is actually helping your brain to stay young. On the other hand, passively taking in information without thinking about it, remembering, and integrating it, will not help to maintain or strengthen cognitive ability.

Learn New Skills

More than a passive receptacle for new information, the brain is designed to put everything it learns to active use. Building new skills, just as you did when you were young, is the best way to maintain brain plasticity. Learning a language, playing an instrument, and taking up hobbies and sports all require continuous practice and progressively higher levels of understanding. The brain is forced to forge new neural paths in order to organize and mobilize various pieces of knowledge. This is plasticity. One good thing about living in the twenty-first century is that serious learning is no longer limited to the young. It has become socially acceptable to be a novice at dancing or sailing at an advanced age, or even to go to college, or start a second or a third career. This is an excellent trend for your brain health, and I urge you to jump on the bandwagon.

Be a People Person

Meaningful involvement in other people's lives not only helps us feel good about ourselves, it exercises the brain, too. Many studies have now shown that people with large and active social networks are far less likely to experience cognitive decline or develop dementia than those who are isolated and have few relationships. When our world shrinks, so does our brain. Stay connected to your family and friends, and extend yourself to include new people and groups into your daily life.

Look Forward to Aging

It's a self-fulfilling prophecy: if you have a positive expectation about your old age, your actual experience is likely to be positive as well. Even though we are bombarded with negative attitudes towards aging, by itself growing old is neither good nor bad. With each passing day, we have at least as much to be grateful for as we do to regret. It all depends on what you make of it, and once again, the choice is yours. The lifestyle changes I have outlined in this book will go a long way towards preserving your natural health and energy. So expect the best for your old age, back up that expectation by taking better and better care of yourself, and you may find a whole new chapter of exciting possibilities opening up in your final years!

Physical Protection

Like any organ, the brain needs to be protected from physical harm. Chronic inflammation damages the brain, causing depression, anxiety, and dementia. Chronic stress triggers a dramatic increase in inflammation. Fluoride in tap water reacts with aluminum in the water to form fluoroaluminum, which causes brain-damaging inflammation. Vaccinations cause brain-damaging inflammation, as do processed oils from the supermarket. Excitotoxins, such as the food additives glutamate (e.g., MSG) and aspartate (e.g., aspartame), also cause inflammatory brain damage.

Antioxidant supplements are helpful in protecting the brain from oxidative damage. These include carotenes and vitamins C and E. Other brain-supporting nutrients include acetyl-L-carnitine, CoQ_{10}, folate, lipoic acid, magnesium, zinc, and vitamins B_1, B_2, B_3, B_6, and B_{12}.

The Bottom Line

- ✓ Your mind can be the greatest healing tool you have, and your best ally for staying healthy and biologically young.

- ✓ Every thought and emotion changes our biochemistry for better or worse. Love, joy, compassion, gratitude, and a sense of purpose promote energy and good health; anger, apathy, loneliness, gloom, and resentment suppress immunity, cause premature aging and undermine health.

✓ Happiness comes from inside, not from externals. Once you make up your mind to be happy, life gets better and easier. One of the greatest gifts you can give yourself is making the choice to be happy.

✓ The mind controls the body, but we control the mind. Although subconscious programming largely determines our mental and physical condition, we have the power to give our subconscious mind new instructions. A strong and clear intention, stated aloud daily, is a way to do this.

✓ Use attention and intention to access your power. In a calm mental and emotional state, pay attention to whatever you would like to change. Then form an intention around what you want it to change into, even if the path is unclear. Know that intention alone has great power to manifest a desired outcome.

✓ Monitor yourself to become aware of automatic negative thoughts and beliefs, and consciously challenge them. Are they really true? Can you turn them around and make them positive?

✓ Stress taxes those parts of the body used to meet emergencies (like adrenals, heart, muscles, and brain) while starving those used for maintenance and repair (like digestive, detoxification, and immune systems). Stress is inflammatory and ages us. We can't always avoid external stressors, but we can minimize their effects. Cultivate a positive "can-do" attitude. Practice taking control where you can and accepting what you can't control. Let go of the past. Develop good friendships that provide mutual support.

✓ Meditation and prayer are time-honored methods for reducing the effects of stress and for cultivating health, harmony, and balance. Scientific studies have shown that both practices improve physical and mental health and extend life expectancy.

✓ Exercise your brain to keep it young. Challenge yourself. Keep learning. Live mindfully in the present, being open to new possibilities and surprises rather than relying on memories and opinions. Stay socially engaged, and expect that aging will be a positive experience.

✓ Protect your brain by avoiding the brain-damaging chemicals fluoride and aluminum in tap water, and excitotoxins like glutamates and aspartame in food. Stay away from processed oils and don't get vaccinations. Include antioxidant supplements like the carotenes, vitamins C and E, acetyl-L-carnitine, CoQ_{10}, lipoic acid, magnesium, zinc, and vitamins B_1, B_2, B_3, B_6, B_{12}, and folate.

CHAPTER 7

The Physical Pathway

Lack of activity destroys the good condition of every human being, while movement and methodical physical exercise save it and preserve it.

—Plato

Exposure to cell phone radiation is the largest human health experiment ever undertaken, without informed consent, and has some 4 billion participants enrolled. . . . I fear we will see a tsunami of brain tumors, although it is too early to see that now since the tumors have a thirty-year latency. I pray I'm wrong, but brace yourself.

—Lloyd Morgan, director of the Central Brain Tumor Registry of the United States, author of *Cell Phones and Brain Tumors: 15 Reasons for Concern*

THE PHYSICAL PATHWAY offers another opportunity to either move yourself toward health, or toward aging and disease. It involves the world of physical factors inside and outside your body. It will lead you to amazing discoveries—for example, how much "free" health benefit you can reap by simply changing the way you breathe or by getting enough sunlight in the right way. It will also give you alarming news about the harmful effects of everyday objects, like the dishwasher in your kitchen and the cell phone in your pocket. Use the Physical Pathway in this chapter the same way as the first three pathways—as a guide to help you make better choices to achieve a healthy and active old age, and to avoid premature aging and disease.

What happens if we persistently use a product in ways it's not designed to be used? In most cases, it will break down a lot faster than if we stick to the recommendations in the owner's manual. That's the headline news behind aging. If we don't move, rest, and use our bodies the way they are meant to be used, we pay with damaged health and accelerated aging. Cars age faster when we drive them off the road or overexpose them to corrosive substances, like road salt. Just as cars are built to run along a smooth surface, our bodies are also best suited to a particular environment. In this chapter, we will cover physical activities, like exercising, breathing, and sleeping, as well as elements of the physical environment—sunlight, noise, and electromagnetic fields—that have a significant impact on health and biological age.

Move Your Body to Stay Young

The benefits of physical exercise extend far beyond flexibility and strength. Physical movement is so fundamental to our nature that when we don't move enough, all of our body chemistry is compromised.

Lack of Exercise Increases Deficiency and Toxicity

Exercise is essential for keeping your cellular energy at high levels, which is essential for health and longevity. As you know by now, your health depends on giving your cells the nutrition they need and protecting them from toxins that can interfere with their normal function. However, here is another factor: *you need to move and stretch your cells.* Moving and stretching cells facilitates the delivery of nutrients and the removal of toxins, addressing both deficiency and toxicity. This is why bedridden people get even sicker. Movement is life. If you aren't moving, you are dying.

Exercise Moves Waste Out of Your Cells

Want proof the human body is designed to move? Consider that one of your body's vital systems—the lymphatic system—does not function well without physical movement. The lymphatic system is your body's sewer, collecting the garbage produced by individual cells and releasing it into your intestines for elimination. It is similar to your circulatory system, which is responsible for delivering nutrients to your cells. But there's a big difference. The circulatory system has a pump—your heart—to keep your blood flowing under pressure to all the cells in your body. The lymphatic system has no such pump. Lymphatic fluids move when you move.

The lymphatic system is a network of capillaries, vessels, and nodes, located near the skin, organs, and major blood veins. Lymphatic fluid carries cellular waste, debris, dead blood cells, pathogens, toxins, and cancer cells out of the tissues. The nodes act as filters, collecting larger pieces of waste to be taken apart by enzymes for easier removal. Every cell in your body consumes nutrients and puts out waste products. Who makes sure that your internal sewer doesn't back up? You do! Every time you use your large muscles—your legs or your arms—you squeeze the lymph vessels and move the lymphatic fluid along. This is one reason why even mild physical exercise will reduce the risk of breast cancer.

Exercise Keeps Your Cells Young

To stay young, you must constantly produce new cells. To produce new cells, you need strong cellular batteries that can store a voltage of –50 mV. *Exercise helps to charge your batteries.* When you exercise, your muscles create a flow of electrons that charge the batteries. Specific activities are better or worse for charging your batteries. Swimming in the ocean or walking barefoot on the beach will donate electrons to you. Swimming in a chlorinated pool will steal electrons from you.

One of the best things you can do to keep yourself healthy and slow the aging process is to adopt a regular exercise routine. Cells accumulate damage as you age due to many factors that often are unavoidable, such as air pollution. The more damaged your cells become, the faster you age and the higher your risk of all kinds of diseases. Interestingly, your body has a mechanism for ridding itself of the damaged parts of cells. This mechanism, called *autophagy*, meaning "self-eating," is like a cellular recycling process. However, autophagy is only activated when the body is under certain kinds of stress, for example, when it's starved. In fact, the healing and rejuvenating effects of fasting, which we discussed in Chapter 5, are due in part to this very phenomenon. Recent research has shown that moderate exercise may also trigger autophagy, helping to keep your cells and your body biologically younger. A 2012 study in *Nature* showed that just thirty minutes of moderate exercise helps renew cells, improve endurance, and facilitate recovery from disease. Dr. Congcong He, one of the authors of the study, said, "Triggering this cellular recycling process is likely a major reason that exercise helps humans boost endurance and ward off diseases."

Exercise Is a Miracle Cure for Aging

In addition to helping deliver nutrients, promoting detoxification, and rejuvenating your cells, exercise directly counteracts three prime causes of aging: chronic inflammation, oxygen deficiency, and depressed immune function. It lowers the amount of inflammatory cytokines in the blood. It provides more oxygen to the tissues. It also stimulates natural killer cell activity, increasing immune function. Exercise also reduces insulin, blood sugar, and IGF (insulin-like growth factor), all of which contribute to inflammation and tumor growth.

Exercise has a powerful effect on the brain. One effect is to promote new brain-cell growth, helping to keep the brain young and in good repair. A 2012 study in *Stroke* found that regular exercise of as little as thirty minutes, three times a week, reduces the risk of dementia and the decline of thinking skills by 60 percent. Exercise also increases levels of serotonin and other important brain chemicals that physically improve brain function and structure. Lack of serotonin causes depression, and studies have found that exercise is better than antidepressant drugs for treating depression.

Exercise Preserves Your Telomeres

Remember telomeres, the tiny units of DNA at the end of each chromosome that shorten each time the cell divides? They maintain genomic stability, prevent DNA damage, and regulate cellular aging. Telomere length is considered a marker of biological age and health. As you get older, your telomeres get shorter and shorter. Eventually, they get too short; the DNA unravels, cell division ceases, and you die. Obesity, psychological stress, and smoking all speed up the telomere-shortening process. Exercise, on the other hand, has been shown to slow down telomere shortening, thus promoting longevity. Recent research has found that the white blood cell telomeres in women who were moderately or highly active were longer than those of sedentary women. Exercise can also protect your telomeres from the damaging effects of stress. A 2010 study in *PLOS ONE* found that: "Vigorous physical activity appears to protect those experiencing high stress by buffering its relationship with telomere length." Among participants who did not exercise, higher levels of stress resulted in telomere shortening. Those who exercised regularly showed no loss of telomere length.

Exercise Prevents Age-Related Muscle Loss

Movement is life, and to move you need healthy muscle tissue. Researchers have discovered that exercise helps preserve your muscles by stimulating muscle stem cells. Mesenchymal stem cells (MSCs) facilitate growth and repair in skeletal muscle. As people age, their muscles become increasingly deficient in MSCs. A 2012 study in *PLOS ONE* concluded that MSCs accumulate in muscle after exercise, promoting growth of new muscle fibers. This study confirms what we already know from experience and common sense: incorporating strength-training throughout life, regardless of your age, is the best strategy to prevent age-related muscle loss. Unfortunately, few people today are acting on this knowledge, with sometimes catastrophic consequences for their health and quality of life. When we do take on the challenge of staying active throughout our lifespan, the results can beat our wildest expectations.

Pace Yourself

While exercise is essential to health and longevity—and most people today don't get enough—some get too much. Extreme exercise can age you just as fast, or even faster, than no exercise. Think of what would happen to the engine of your car if you drove it at 120 miles per hour every single day. When the body is pushed to the limit, all metabolic activity speeds up, which, in turn, releases floods of free radicals, damaging the organs and tissues. Sustaining extreme effort for hours, as do marathon runners and triathletes, for example, depletes the body of its reserves and compromises cellular repairs. When this happens routinely, cumulative damage can show up quickly as premature aging, chronic health problems, or even premature death. If extreme sports are your thing, you need to rethink what you are doing, and at least take special care with diet and supplements to help compensate.

Yeah . . . But Where Do I Find the Time?

Historically, getting the physical activity necessary for good health was not a problem because meeting our basic needs required a lot of movement. Now, however, we are the most sedentary people in history, and our health is failing. All exercise is good, whether it is walking, swimming, or tennis, but many people say they can't find the time to do it. Here is a form of exercise that takes very little time.

Rebounding

Not a big fan of huffing and puffing? Wish you could take an "exercise pill" instead? Fortunately, there is a way to cheat. Rebounding is a unique form of exercise that involves bouncing up and down on a mini-trampoline—and its effects are almost magical. It is simple, surprisingly easy to do, safe, and a lot of fun. Best of all, just about anyone can do it, right at home, regardless of age or physical condition. You can even rebound while you watch the evening news or talk on the telephone. Rebounding tones, conditions, strengthens, and heals the entire body in as little as fifteen minutes per day, although more is better.

How does it do all that? Jumping up and down on a rebounder moves and stretches every cell in your body simultaneously, so it is a concentrated form of exercise. As a result, your entire body (internal organs, bones, connective tissue, and skin) becomes stronger, more flexible, and healthier. Blood circulation, oxygen delivery, lymphatic drainage, and toxin removal are vastly improved. Visualize for a moment holding a balloon filled with water and notice how gravity pulls on the water, slightly stretching the balloon. If you moved the balloon rapidly up and down, the extra gravitational force would cause the balloon to significantly stretch and distort. When you bounce up and down on a rebounder, this is what happens to every cell in your body. Rebounding alternately puts pressure on and takes pressure off the cells, like squeezing a sponge. This moving and stretching of the cells facilitates nutrient delivery and toxin removal, which is exactly what you need to be healthy. Amazingly, you get all of this benefit without going to the gym, working up a sweat, or ending up with sore muscles and possible injuries. One caveat is that poor-quality rebounders may shock the joints and tissues and cause injury. Look for barrel springs that are fatter in the middle and tapered at the ends.

Stephanie's Story

Consider the effects of rebounding exercise on Stephanie, the fifty-six-year-old overweight mother of three who was suffering from depressed immunity, experiencing frequent ear infections, sore throats, and many allergies. She also suffered from poor digestion, shoulder pain, a bad back, and a painful knee, the result of an accident and subsequent knee surgery. Stephanie was tired of feeling sick. On my advice, she took up rebounding to get some exercise.

Within two weeks of rebounding only fifteen minutes a day, Stephanie saw positive changes in her body. The first thing she noticed was her skin becoming tighter and toned, including on her face. As she continued exercising, her cellulite began to disappear, as did the spider veins in her legs. The neck tension and shoulder pain that used to build as she worked on her computer was completely relieved. Stephanie increased her exercise time to two fifteen-minute sessions per day. She began to lose weight, her allergies cleared up, and the earaches and sore throats stopped happening. Her skin was clear and glowing. Her digestion improved. Her back felt better; her knee strengthened and was no longer painful.

Stephanie's life was better, and all it took was a moderate amount of high-quality exercise. She has now lengthened her exercise time to an hour a day, and she claims she has discovered "the fountain of youth." Rebounding is almost like a wonder drug.

One-Minute Eye Yoga

Declining vision and other eye problems are common first signs of aging in our society. There is a good reason for it. The human eye is designed to look far into the distance. Our ancestors would not have survived in the wild without long-range vision. However, modern living makes long vistas less common, with a significant portion of our time spent indoors, where we engage in close-range activities like reading, writing, working on the computer, or watching TV. This emphasis on short-range focus unnaturally strains the eyes. The artificial light and the glare from the computer, cell phone, and TV screens don't help matters either. What can you do? The answer is astonishingly simple: exercise your eye muscles! When working on the computer, take a break every hour to change your eye focus. Look up, look down, look out of the window and far ahead, roll your eyes to the left, to the right, and trace a figure eight with your eyeballs. Do this while waiting in line and when stuck in traffic. Get used to feeling the strain in your eyes and relieving it with the simple eye stretches I have just described. You'd be surprised how much eye trouble you will save yourself down the road. For more information on eye exercises, see Appendix C.

Breathing

Oxygen is our most critical nutrient. It is used by cells to create the energy we need to stay alive—you can only live minutes without it. Just as you can control what foods you eat, the toxins you are exposed to, the thoughts you put into your mind, and how much exercise you get, you can also control how you breathe and how much oxygen you supply to your body. The way you breathe directly impacts your resistance to disease and can substantially affect how you look and feel, and even how long you live. Correct breathing goes a long way toward keeping you healthy, relaxed, and mentally alert.

Lack of Oxygen Causes Premature Aging

The latest scientific research concludes that premature aging is in large part caused by lack of oxygen. Oxygen deficiency in the human body has been linked to every major illness, including cancer, diabetes, respiratory disease, and heart disease, as well as muscle aches, forgetfulness, heart palpitations, circulatory or digestive problems, excessive colds and infections, and all of the visible signs of aging—gray hair, wrinkles, pale complexion, and so on. Oxygen displaces harmful free radicals, neutralizes environmental toxins, and destroys infectious bacteria, parasites, microbes, and viruses. It is vital for our brain function. It calms the mind and stabilizes the nervous system. Without oxygen, nothing works very well—or at all.

Healthy arteries and capillaries make it easier for the blood to carry oxygen to the cells. Exercise improves circulation and speeds up oxygen delivery. However, a very important factor in supplying oxygen to your cells is how you normally breathe. Deep breathing equals more oxygen, and shallow breathing equals less. For most of us, our breathing is way too shallow.

What Is Overbreathing?

We were all born knowing how to breathe. However, the stress of modern living has caused many people to develop poor breathing habits. The most common problem is shallow or rapid breathing, also called overbreathing. Despite the name, overbreathing actually results in less oxygen being available to cells. Overbreathing is usually caused by stress, and it manifests as shallow chest breathing, irregular breathing, rapid breathing, or holding of the breath. On occasion, overbreathing is not a problem, and we all do it at times. However, for most of us, overbreathing has become the norm—just as sustained low-grade anxiety, dissatisfaction, and mental stress have become the norm.

Overbreathing causes constriction of the blood vessels. This can result in up to a 50 percent reduction of oxygen and glucose to the brain—immediately affecting one's ability to learn, think, remember, and perform physically. Many people feel dizzy or light-headed when stressed, due to oxygen shortage. Oxygen shortage at the cellular level produces numerous side effects, including heart palpitations, irregular heartbeat, dizziness, muscle spasms, muscle fatigue, high blood pressure, poor memory, asthma attacks, poor concentration, anxiety, and other symptoms.

Overbreathing not only takes in too little oxygen, it also expels too much carbon dioxide. This is a problem because the body uses carbon dioxide to regulate oxygen delivery. Oxygen is transported to tissues by bonding with hemoglobin in red blood cells. Normal oxygen metabolism creates carbon dioxide as a waste product. When local concentrations of carbon dioxide are high, this signals the red blood cells to release their oxygen so that your cells can obtain a new supply of oxygen. When you expel too much carbon dioxide through rapid breathing, there is insufficient carbon dioxide present to cause the hemoglobin to release its oxygen. Your cells and tissues then become oxygen deficient. Another problem with breathing out too fast is that your blood ends up with too little acid-forming carbon dioxide, which causes the pH of your blood to become too alkaline. While cells can become too acidic or alkaline and still live, your blood must always be kept in a very narrow range. To rebalance blood pH, the body takes alkaline minerals out of the blood and dumps them in the urine. The chronic loss of alkaline minerals, such as calcium and magnesium, creates a deficiency of alkaline minerals in the cells, making the cells acidic. Acidic cells compromise your ability to obtain and use oxygen, creating a deficiency of oxygen respiration—a prescription for cancer. Over-breathing, combined with an acidic diet, makes cells too acidic, damaging your cell batteries and accelerating the aging process.

Breathe Right

To breathe correctly, it is important to bring air down into the lungs by using the diaphragm, a deep abdominal muscle that nature intended for breathing. Breathing downward with the diaphragm (belly breathing) is an effortless and efficient way to breathe. Instead, people often use their chest and upper back to breathe (chest breathing), which takes more effort and provides less oxygen. Breathing downward (as opposed to outward with the chest) moves the viscera (guts) down and away, making more room for the lungs. This creates the capacity for more air in your lungs and more oxygen for your tissues, whether you are exercising or at rest. Each breath should begin down in the belly, only moving up into the chest at the end.

Correct breathing should be effortless, through the nose rather than the mouth, and relatively slow—at a resting rate of less than fifteen breaths per minute, preferably eight to ten. Here is a simple test to check how you are doing: Relax and count the number of breaths you take per minute. What you want is to learn to breathe with the diaphragm and keep the number of breaths per minute to less than fifteen and preferably less than ten. The key word is "effortless." Let your body do the breathing for you, as it was designed to do.

During aerobic exercise, keep the breath down in the belly and out of the chest as much as possible. Breathing has such profound effects, both physically and psychologically, it is little surprise that many ancient traditions—such as meditation, yoga, and martial arts—rely first and foremost on breathing technique. Daily deep-breathing exercises are very calming, and they will help keep you oxygenated and healthy.

Are You Getting Enough Sun?

Sunlight is one of nature's most powerful healing agents, yet we are repeatedly advised to avoid it. This bad advice to stay out of the sun has cost countless thousands of lives by perpetrating an epidemic of vitamin D deficiency. Low vitamin D levels are a causative factor in heart disease, multiple sclerosis, osteoporosis, Type 1 diabetes, infections, autoimmune diseases, depression, asthma, and cancer. Science doesn't even begin to understand all the marvelous benefits of sunlight, yet the disease industry continues to perpetuate the myth that the sun ages your skin and causes cancer. Exactly the opposite is true. Cells have light-activated receptors that, when triggered, initiate a number of beneficial and cancer-protective biological reactions. Scientists are beginning to examine whether the acupuncture meridians function as a photon transfer system, resembling fiber optics, delivering sunlight throughout the body.

Get 90 Percent of Your Vitamin D from Sunlight

Vitamin D is one of our most important nutrients, and we were designed to manufacture up to 90 percent of it through the interaction of sunlight with cholesterol-like compounds in our skin. If sunlight were bad for us, why would Mother Nature make us dependent on it? Our bodies need sunlight, and we are missing it badly. More than 40 percent of the American population is deficient in vitamin D, and that goes up to about 60 percent by the end of the winter. One reason influenza spreads so quickly in the winter is because people are vitamin D deficient, and vitamin D is crucial to immune function. The best time of day to get your vitamin D is two hours before or after noon. You don't need a flu shot; you probably just need more vitamin D!

Sunlight Nourishes Your Whole Body

Modern research shows that sunlight nourishes and energizes the human body and helps prevent infections from bacteria, molds, and viruses. Sunlight enhances the immune system by increasing white blood cell count, as well as gamma globulin, a protein that helps the body fight infection. Significantly, sunlight stimulates the production of red blood cells, increasing the oxygen content of the blood. Sunlight is also good for the heart. It enables the body to lower the resting pulse rate, lower blood pressure, and lower cholesterol and triglycerides. In fact, sunlight can decrease cholesterol by more than 30 percent. Sunlight also enhances the power of the skin to resist diseases such as psoriasis, eczema, and acne. It also lowers blood sugar and enhances liver function. It stimulates the liver to produce an enzyme that increases your ability to detoxify environmental pollutants. Further, sunlight stimulates the pineal gland to produce vital brain chemicals such as tryptamines, which cheer you up and prevent anxiety and depression.

Do not use sunscreens. Sunscreens block essential wavelengths for vitamin D production. Even worse, most sunscreen products have toxic and even carcinogenic ingredients. Dating from antiquity, high-quality olive oil or coconut oil has been used to protect against sun damage. Put it on your skin before and after you go out in the sun. However, the low quality olive and coconut oils sold in most stores will not do the job.

. . . But Don't Overdo It

Caution: This is not an invitation to rush out and get sunburned. Sunburn damages DNA and can cause cancer. Too much of a good thing can be bad for you. People with light skin need less sunlight than those with dark skin. In fact, people with dark skin need a lot more sunlight to get the same benefits. Use the sun sensibly. Don't abuse it, and it will be your partner in health. If your skin starts getting pink, get out of the sun; you have already had more than you should. It is best to get sun as often as possible in small, graduated doses. When you are outdoors for long periods, wear protective clothing and a wide-brimmed hat. If you eat a fresh, plant-based diet that is rich in antioxidants and essential fatty acids, this will provide enormous natural protection from the sun. Carotenes are known to be very protective. The processed oils and foods that most people eat, on the other hand, will accelerate sun damage.

Electromagnetic Fields

Most of us are aware of the chemical pollution in our environment, but few appreciate the extent and impact of electromagnetic pollution. There is a growing body of evidence indicating that brain cancer is only one of the many health problems produced by our new wireless society. Invisible to the human eye, electromagnetic fields (EMFs) are present everywhere in our environment. The human body is itself electromagnetic, and its electrical system, which relays nerve signals and stimulates heartbeats, is affected by the external EMFs coming from Wi-Fi networks, cordless phones, cell phones, cell phone towers, and even home electric meters. Over the last century, exposure to man-made EMFs has been increasing steadily, as growing demand for electricity, ever-advancing technologies, and changes in social behavior have created more and more artificial sources. At home and at work, from the generation and transmission of electricity to domestic appliances and industrial equipment to telecommunications and broadcasting, all of us are now exposed to a complex mix of electrical and magnetic fields.

Your Body Is Electromagnetically Sensitive

The human body is an electromagnetic device, and it produces its own weak electromagnetic field. Cell membranes act as capacitors to store voltage; they also act as semiconductors, diodes, and microprocessors that control cell function by interacting with the environment. No one who understands the physics of the human body would even question the fact that we are affected by external electromagnetic fields. The real questions are about the nature of these effects, how long they last, and how harmful they might be. The effects of EMFs are difficult to study; there are so many variables involved. However, you need to be aware of at least some of what is known.

Increasingly, people are becoming affected by external electromagnetic fields. It is estimated that 3 to 8 percent of the population in developed countries now experience serious electrohypersensitivity symptoms, while 35 percent experience mild symptoms. Some people can be totally debilitated just by walking into a Wi-Fi-equipped area. One symptom of electrohypersensitivity is altered sugar metabolism similar to diabetes. In fact, some researchers believe we even have a new kind of diabetes caused by electromagnetic sensitivity. A groundbreaking study in a 2010 *European Journal of Oncology* found that cordless phones can interfere with the heart, causing abnormal rhythms. Dr. Thomas Rau, medical director of the world-renowned Paracelsus Clinic in Switzerland, said in an interview at *www.ElectromagneticHealth.org* that he is convinced that electromagnetic loads lead to concentration problems, ADHD, tinnitus, migraines, insomnia, arrhythmia, Parkinson's, and cancer.

High-Voltage Power Lines Increase Cancer Risk

A 2007 study in the *Internal Medicine Journal* looked at a database of 850 patients diagnosed with lymphatic and bone-marrow cancers between 1972 and 1980. The study found that living next to high-voltage power lines increased the risk of cancer. People who lived within 328 yards of a power line up to age five were five times more likely to develop cancer. In addition, children who lived that close to a power line at any point during the first fifteen years of their lives were three times more likely to develop cancer as adults. The study concluded that living for a prolonged period near high-voltage power lines is likely to increase the risk of leukemia, lymphoma, and related conditions later in life. The power industry had dismissed safety concerns after previous short-term studies failed to show a link. *This 2007 study is significant because it proves that the cancer shows up, not right away, but much later in adults who were exposed as children.* Obviously, these are long-lasting effects. Based on this study and others, it would be prudent not to live, work, or go to school within 300 yards of a high-voltage power line.

EMFs in Our Daily Living

We are all exposed to EMFs in our daily living. We can't escape them. Electromagnetic pollution is the single-largest change we have made to our environment. Cell phones, computer screens, TV sets, hair dryers, refrigerators, dishwashers, and even the clock radio by the side of your bed are putting out unhealthy levels of EMFs. Driving your car exposes you to a lot of EMFs. While we have little personal control over many of the EMFs in our environment, such as radio and TV broadcasts, we have a great deal of control over some of them. Cell phone use is one example. A Swedish study in a 2006 issue of *International Archives of Occupational and Environmental Health* found that heavy users of cell phones had a 240 percent increase in brain tumors on the side of their head on which the phone was used. The study defined heavy use as more than 2,000 total hours, or approximately one hour of use per workday, for ten years. This is a good reason to limit cell phone use and to use the speakerphone option to avoid holding the phone next to your head. In 2007, the European Environment Agency, the official environmental watchdog of the European Union, warned that cell phone technology "could lead to a health crisis similar to those caused by asbestos, smoking, and lead in petrol."

Cell Phones Are Threatening Our Young

Tragically, more and more children and teens are using cell phones. In the United States, nine out of ten sixteen-year-olds have their own cell phones, as do many primary school children. It is noteworthy that brain cancer has now surpassed leukemia as the number-one cancer killer in children. The incidence of pediatric brain cancers in Australia has increased 21 percent in just one decade.

Because the negative effects of cell phone usage are not immediate, people think cell phones are safe. Cell phones have been used heavily for less than twenty years, but it can take up to thirty years for brain tumors to develop as a result of their use. Children, however, are more susceptible, because their cells are reproducing more rapidly. Their brains and nervous systems are still developing, and their skulls are thinner. A 2007 study in *Occupational and Environmental Medicine* by Dr. Lennart Hardell, a professor in oncology and cancer epidemiology in Sweden, found that teenagers with heavy use of cell phones have 500 percent more brain cancer as young adults. Surprisingly, young people who used the cordless phones found in many homes had almost as much risk—more than 400 percent higher than the control group. In Europe and the United Kingdom, the incidence of brain tumors has increased by 40 percent over the last twenty years. Some researchers are predicting an epidemic of brain cancer as cell phone use continues to grow.

Cell Phones Threaten All of Us

Adding to our concerns, Israeli scientist Dr. Siegal Sadetzki concluded in a study published in a 2008 issue of the *American Journal of Epidemiology* that there is a link between cell phone usage and the development of cancer of the salivary glands. Heavy cell phone users were found to have an increased risk of about 50 percent for developing a tumor of the main salivary gland, compared to those who did not use cell phones. Other studies have indicated risks beyond brain and salivary tumors, finding cognitive problems, disorientation, eye damage, bone damage, Alzheimer's, and other risks.

Research sponsored by the telecommunications industry found an almost 300 percent increase in the incidence of genetic damage when human blood cells were exposed to cell phone radiation. Dr.

Ronald B. Herberman, the head of the University of Pittsburgh Cancer Institute, has testified before the U.S. House Subcommittee on Domestic Policy that regular cell phone use doubles the risk of brain cancer. After reviewing the existing data, Dr. Herberman now advises against using cell phones in public places because it exposes other people to the hazardous EMFs that you are generating. Cell phones not only affect the user, but like secondhand smoke, also affect those around us. Children especially should be protected from EMF pollution. Do not use cell phones in close proximity to children. In 2009, Dr. Herberman issued an unprecedented warning to his faculty and staff: *Limit cell phone use because of the health risks.*

The same goes for Bluetooth devices and unshielded headsets. According to Dr. Vini Khurana, an associate professor of neuro-surgery at the Australian National University who has studied the link between mobile phones and malignant brain tumors, these could "convert the user's head into an effective, potentially self-harming antenna."

Living Close to Cell Phone Towers Damages Your Health

German researchers reporting in a 2004 issue of *Umwelt Medizin Gesellschaft* found that people living within 1,200 feet of a cell tower experienced high cancer rates and developed their tumors on average eight years earlier than the national average. Breast cancer topped the list. Spanish researchers reporting in a 2003 issue of *Biology and Medicine* found that people living within 1,000 feet of cellular antennas developed illnesses at average power densities of only 0.11 to 0.19 microwatts per centimeter, which is thousands of times lower than those allowed by international exposure standards. Researchers in Israel reported in a 2004 issue of *International Journal of Cancer Prevention* that people who lived near a cell tower for three to seven years had a cancer rate four times higher than the control population. People living close to cell phone towers suffer extreme sleep disruption, chronic fatigue, nausea, skin problems, irritability, brain disturbances, and cardiovascular problems.

There Is No Such Thing as "Free" Wi-Fi

Rooftop transmitters, which readily pass microwave radiation into structures, can be especially dangerous. Across the world, there are reports of cancer clusters and extreme illness in office and apartment buildings where antennas are placed. In 2006, the top floors of a University of Melbourne office building were closed after a brain tumor cluster drew media attention to the risks of microwave communications transmitters on top of the building. Radiation in living spaces near cell phone transmitters has been measured at up to 65 microwatts per square centimeter; the FCC's maximum safety limit is 580 microwatts, so people are told the cell towers are safe. However, this can't be true. The Spanish researchers above found problems at 0.11 to 0.19 microwatts, and remember that during the Cold War, the Soviets bombarded the U.S. Embassy in Moscow with a constant 0.01 microwatts of microwave radiation. This made international news because of all the health problems it caused at the embassy.

Countless Wi-Fi systems, both indoors and out, accommodate wireless laptop computers, personal digital assistants, Wi-Fi-enabled phones, gaming devices, video cameras, even parking and utility meters. Hundreds of cities already have or are planning to fund Wi-Fi networks, each consisting of thousands of small microwave transmitters bolted to buildings, street lamps, park benches, bus stops, and even buried under sidewalks. All this has been planned with virtually no studies or warnings about radiation exposure. Not a single environmental or public health study has been required as the industry unleashes this new wireless technology from which no living thing will escape.

Dr. Robert Becker, author of *The Body Electric: Electromagnetism and the Foundation of Life*, is noted for his decades of research on the effects of electromagnetic pollution. He warns, "Even if we survive the chemical and atomic threats to our existence, there is the strong possibility that increasing electropollution could set in motion irreversible changes leading to our extinction before we are even aware of them."

What You Can Do to Protect Yourself from EMFs

Cell phones are a fact of life. They aren't going away. The challenge is to use them sensibly. Limit your cell phone use to only the most essential calls, and then limit the call to less than two minutes. When cell phones are on they are emitting radiation, even when you are not using them; do not carry a cell phone close to your body while it is on. Keep your phone turned off when it is not being used;

turn it on as needed to check for messages. Do not hold a phone next to your brain. Use the speakerphone feature to make your calls, and keep the phone as far away as possible. Keep infants and young children away from the immediate vicinity when you make a call. Do not allow children under the age of eighteen to use a cell phone except in emergencies, or at least strongly advise them how to minimize the dangers involved, like by using the speakerphone.

Use of cell phones inside buildings, cars, or airplanes increases your exposure, because it increases the radiation a phone must emit in order to function. Don't live within 1,200 feet of a cell phone antenna. Text messaging can reduce, but not eliminate, health risk. The evidence is becoming overwhelming that cell phone use is hazardous to your health, but do not count on the government to protect you. Federal exposure limits have been deliberately set so high that, no matter how much additional wireless radiation is added to the national burden, it will always be "within standards."

When buying a home or choosing an apartment, choose one that is not adjacent to high-voltage transmission lines, cell phone towers, or transformers. Be prudent in the use of appliances. When possible, use rechargeable battery-powered appliances rather than plug-in models. Do not stand next to an electrical appliance when it is turned on, especially for an extended time. Turn on the dishwasher in the kitchen after you've finished your tasks and are ready to leave the room. Avoid electric blankets or use them only to warm up the bed before you get in. Keep telephones, answering machines, and electric clocks away from your head while you are sleeping. Increase distance from televisions (at least six feet away), and avoid appliances that come into close contact with your body, such as hairdryers and plug-in electric razors.

Radiation

Technically, radiation means energy particles or waves that travel outward in all directions (radiate) from a source. Radio waves, heat, and visible light are all examples of radiation. All radiation brings changes to the living organisms through which it passes; some are beneficial and others are harmful. The man-made electromagnetic fields and microwaves that I discussed above are examples of harmful radiation that is nonionizing, meaning it does not carry enough energy to disrupt molecular bonds and convert atoms into ions.

Radiation with sufficient energy to ionize atoms is called ionizing radiation. This type of radiation, found in atomic bombs, medical radiation, and X-rays, is what most people think of when they hear the word "*radiation.*" Ionizing radiation is far more dangerous to living organisms than nonionizing radiation. The ions that are produced by ionizing radiation, even at low radiation powers, can damage cells and DNA. As you know, DNA mutations contribute to aging and a host of diseases, including cancer. While there are limits within which nonionizing radiation is considered "safe," no level of ionizing radiation is ever safe. Therefore, you need to be aware of your exposure and understand your options.

Ionizing Radiation Accelerates Aging

Since the Chernobyl catastrophe of 1986, scientists have been studying its effects on humans. Numerous studies in Russia, Belarus, and Ukraine show that decline in health brought about by ionizing radiation mimics the normal process of aging. In their report "Does Ionizing Radiation Accelerate the Aging Phenomena?" presented at the 2006 international conference "Twenty Years After the Chernobyl Accident: Future Outlook," Ukrainian scientists Vladimir Bebeshko and others wrote, "Ionizing radiation influences both cell structure and cell function at molecular and genetic levels. The effects of ionizing radiation on cells and cellular changes are the same or similar to biological mechanisms at work during the normal aging process: reactions of free radicals, the DNA repair process, changes in the functioning of the immune system, changed mechanisms in fat metabolism, [and] systemic changes to the nerve system."

Studies of Japanese atomic bomb survivors showed that life expectancy following ionizing radiation was significantly shortened by noncancerous diseases. Recent research from Russia, Belarus, and Ukraine found that degenerative diseases among survivors occurred ten to fifteen years earlier than they did among the general population. Survivors typically experience accelerated aging of blood vessels in the brain and the coronary vessels, senile cataracts, arteriosclerosis of the eye blood vessels, and loss of the higher intellectual cognitive functions.

Look Out for Radioactivity in the Environment

We have no control over about half of the ionizing radiation in our lives, because it comes from natural sources. Our soil, water, and air are all contaminated to a greater or lesser degree by radioactive fallouts from nuclear plants and other industries around the world. The aftereffects of nuclear disasters, like the 1986 Chernobyl incident and the 2011 explosion of the Fukushima Daiichi nuclear power plant in Japan, are long-lasting and widespread. For example, because of the radioactive fallout from Chernobyl, the infant mortality rate in Germany, Denmark, Iceland, Latvia, Norway, Poland, Sweden, and Hungary increased between 1987 and 1992 by 8.8 percent. Similarly, mortality rates increased on the West Coast of the United States following the radioactive contamination from the Japanese explosions. Certain industries, such as phosphate mining in Florida, also create radioactive fallouts. You can measure the level of radiation in the ground and water where you live. If your local ambient radiation is high, you might want to consider a different home. At least, avoid drinking contaminated water and use ventilation to remove radioactive gas (radon) from your basement. While being exposed, take antioxidants to counter the increased production of health-damaging free radicals. Radioactive iodine is one of the most common radioactive elements in the environment. If you are exposed to radioactive iodine, take iodine supplements to supply the body with healthy iodine.

Shy Away from X-Ray Machines

We do have a lot of control over the other half of the ionizing radiation we are exposed to—that which comes from man-made devices, primarily medical X-rays. Seemingly "benign" dental X-rays and other radiological procedures can subject the body to significant physical harm. Given that most diagnostic X-rays, including mammograms, are not medically necessary, we should consider them health risks rather than something helpful. Carefully evaluate the potential harm against any possible benefits (see more about medical X-rays in Chapter 9, "The Medical Pathway").

Another ubiquitous source of X-ray radiation is airport scanners. In a 2010 interview with Agence France-Presse, a French news agency, Dr. Michael Love, a radiation expert at Johns Hopkins University School of Medicine, had this to say: "No exposure to X-rays is considered beneficial. We know X-rays are hazardous, but we have a situation at the airports where people are so eager to fly that they will risk their lives in this manner." To protect yourself, you can decline going through the scanner and request a manual search instead.

Sleep

Getting a good night's sleep is essential to health and another piece of the puzzle to prevent and reverse premature aging. The body is designed for certain sleep patterns, and disturbing those patterns can seriously alter the balance of hormones in your body. The reality is the body has been programmed over millennia to sleep when it's dark and be awake during daylight. This is how our ancestors lived. If you do otherwise, you are sending conflicting signals to the body, upsetting its normal biochemistry. The more you deviate, the greater the negative impact.

The necessary amount of sleep varies from person to person. Some people do quite well on just a few hours of sleep, while others barely function without getting a full ten hours. Most people need between seven and nine hours. Research indicates that, for the majority of us, sleeping less than eight hours a night has significant cumulative consequences. A 2004 study by Harvard Medical School of more than 82,000 nurses participating in the Nurses' Health Study found that getting less than six hours of sleep per night increases the risk of premature death. Links have also been discovered between too little sleep and diabetes, obesity, hypertension, and high cholesterol.

The emerging picture is that not sleeping enough, being awake in the early-morning hours, or waking up frequently during the night throws the body's internal clock out of whack. "Lack of sleep disrupts every physiologic function in the body," said Dr. Eve Van Cauter of the University of Chicago in an October 9, 2005, article in the *Washington Post*. She went on to say, "We have nothing in our biology that allows us to adapt to this behavior."

Obey Your Biological Clock

While humans are the only species capable of manufacturing timekeeping devices, *circadian rhythms* or the "biological clocks" are common to all life on the planet. A biological clock is encoded in our genes. It is attuned to the twenty-four-hour day, and it sets in motion all cyclical processes in the cells, including hormone production and DNA repair, based on the regular cycles of light, dark, and sleep. Science had long known that normal functioning of the biological clock is linked to neurological health, without understanding the precise cause-and-effect relationship between the two. In 2011, a study in *Neurobiology and Disease* proved that disruption of circadian rhythms can cause neurodegeneration, loss of motor function, and premature death. In humans, disrupted clock mechanisms are linked to aging and neurologic disorders like Alzheimer's and Huntington's disease. Neurodegeneration, in turn, causes more damage to the clock function. A healthy biological clock, on the other hand, protects the brain and the nervous system, preventing premature aging.

Unfortunately, a good night's sleep is increasingly losing out to late-night TV, the Internet, and other distractions of modern life. According to a poll by the National Sleep Foundation, the majority of Americans are not getting enough sleep. Only 40 percent of the respondents reported getting a good night's sleep every night, or almost every night. Lawrence Epstein, past president of the American Academy of Sleep Medicine and author of *The Harvard Medical School Guide to a Good Night's Sleep,* said, "We have in our society this idea that you can just get by without sleep or manipulate when you sleep without any consequences. What we're finding is that's just not true."

Insufficient Sleep Disrupts Hormonal Balance

Sleep regulates hormone production. Hormone balance is essential to health and affects the rate at which you age. Studies indicate that lack of sleep increases the production of stress hormones, such as cortisol. Cortisol helps regulate the release of disease-battling natural killer cells, but too much cortisol will throw the immune system out of balance. Night-shift workers and people who wake up frequently during the night are more likely to suffer from abnormal cortisol rhythms that interfere with the body's ability to self-regulate and self-repair.

Melatonin is another hormone affected by sleep. Melatonin interferes with tumor growth and protects against cancer. Melatonin also has antioxidant properties that help protect DNA and prevent aging. The brain produces this hormone during sleep. Melatonin production is sensitive to the amount of light we are exposed to and the amount of sleep we get. Shift workers who are up all night produce less melatonin. But you don't need to work the night shift in order to upset your melatonin balance. The light-producing electrical gadgets that are now increasingly part of our lives are increasingly upsetting that balance. Too many people keep these devices in their bedroom and are continually exposed to light during sleep. Research shows that even the smallest amount of light from the LEDs of iPods, laptops, electronic readers, and TV sets is sufficient to cut melatonin production in half. *To get good quality sleep you must sleep in a totally dark room.* Insufficient melatonin affects levels of other hormones, increasing estrogen levels. High estrogen increases the risk of breast and prostate cancer. When melatonin production is reduced by artificial light sources, our nighttime rhythms are disturbed, and normal cellular repair is disrupted. This results in repair deficits and aging. As a rule, the body requires seven to nine hours of uninterrupted sleep each night, with no light distraction, to complete the repair functions that are essential to maintaining optimal health.

Poor Sleep Habits Promote Inflammation

Interfering with the body's natural rhythms is never a good idea—health can only occur when the body is balanced and functioning normally. Because sleep helps to restore the body's internal environment, people who sleep poorly or do not get enough sleep have higher levels of inflammation. People who get six or fewer hours of sleep typically measure higher levels of inflammatory markers such as IL-6 (interleukin-6) and C-reactive protein.

Cell Phones Make Strange Bedfellows

Cell phones are another problem affecting sleep. An international study published in the 2007 *Progress in Electromagnetics Research Symposium Proceedings* said there was now "more than sufficient evidence" to show that cell phone radiation delays and reduces sleep. Using cell phones before bed causes people to take longer to reach the deeper stages of sleep and to spend less time in these stages. Lack of deep sleep interferes with the body's ability to do its daily repairs. The resulting repair deficits accelerate the aging process, as well as impair your immune system, leaving you less able to fight off diseases of all kinds.

Sound Sleep Prevents Alzheimer's

A good night's sleep protects against memory loss and Alzheimer's disease, which presently ranks as the sixth-leading cause of death in the United States. A 2012 study presented at the *American Academy of Neurology* found that the quality and duration of sleep may affect memory function and the risk of Alzheimer's disease later in life. Disrupted sleep appears to be associated with the buildup of amyloid plaques—a marker of Alzheimer's—in the brains of people without memory problems. The researchers found that those who did not wake up frequently during the night were five times less likely to possess the amyloid plaque buildup compared to those who slept poorly or less than seven hours in total. Apparently, the amyloid protein clumps and tangles that occur as a normal process of metabolism in the brain are cleared during sleep, but the sleep has to last from seven to nine hours.

How to Sleep for Good Health

Your sleep needs are individual to you, and you may require more or less sleep than someone of the same age, gender, and activity level. Listen to your body. To determine how much you need, make note of how you feel immediately upon awakening. If you still feel tired, you probably need more sleep. The first step in getting a good night's sleep is allowing yourself to do it. Stress is well known to interfere with sleep, and if you lose sleep, you won't be able to handle stress as well. This can lead to more stress and more loss of sleep in a vicious cycle.

Try going to bed by 10:00 PM in a dark and quiet room and get a good eight hours of sleep. The body recharges the adrenal glands between 11:00 PM and 1:00 AM, which helps to balance your hormones, so you should be asleep during those hours. Adequate sleep is one of the most important factors in your health and quality of life.

Noise

Chronic noise disrupts normal hormone balance and immune response, and creates inflammation in the body. Noise has also been linked to aging through disrupted sleep patterns and the resulting hormonal imbalances. Research has proven that noise can cause health damage far beyond sleep loss. For example, workers chronically exposed to loud noise suffered calcium and magnesium losses, which can result in a variety of health problems from osteoporosis to cancer. The body reacts to noise by secreting inflammatory chemicals (cytokines), resulting in DNA damage and aging. Some researchers believe that one reason cytokine production rises as we grow older is exposure to a lifetime of noise.

We have created a society where noise is normal. This is just one of the fundamental changes we have made in our modern world, and it is costing us our health. As much as possible, reduce the amount of noise in your life.

The Bottom Line

✓ Movement is so fundamental to our nature that healthy cell chemistry is compromised without it. Moving and stretching cells rejuvenates them and helps them to absorb nutrients and eliminate toxins. Exercise counteracts three primary causes of aging: chronic inflammation, oxygen deficiency, and weakened immunity.

✓ Bouncing on a high-quality rebounder is the easiest and most efficient form of exercise. Rebounding tones, conditions, strengthens, and heals the entire body in as little as fifteen minutes a day. More is even better.

✓ Our vision deteriorates when our eyes are used continuously for short-range vision. To change focus and reduce eyestrain, take one-minute breaks from computer work or reading every hour and give your eyes the short workout described in this chapter.

✓ Tension and stress cause rapid, shallow "chest-breathing." This creates oxygen deficiency, which is linked to many symptoms and diseases, as well as with accelerated aging. "Belly-breathing," in which the abdomen expands and contracts naturally and without effort, supplies needed oxygen as well as relaxation and a sense of calm. Time your breathing for one minute. There should be less than fifteen complete breaths per minute; less than ten is even better.

✓ While we are told that sunlight is bad for us and causes skin aging and cancer, the opposite is true. Sunlight benefits health and curbs aging in a host of ways, as long as you do not overdo it. If your skin turns pink, get out of the sun. Get sun often, but in small, graduated doses, so you build up a protective tan. Where necessary, wear protective clothing and a wide-brimmed hat. Get plenty of protective antioxidants, especially the carotenes. Many cultures rub olive oil or coconut oil into the skin before and during sun exposure. Eating processed oils and processed foods, however, will accelerate sun damage.

✓ Electromagnetic fields (EMFs) generated by electrical appliances, Wi-Fi networks, cell phones, cordless phones, cell phone towers, and high-voltage power lines, have been insufficiently studied. However, what we do know is alarming enough to warrant limiting exposures, especially for children. Follow the rules for using cell phones given in this chapter. If possible, avoid living adjacent to high-voltage transmission lines, cell phone towers, or transformers. Use battery-powered appliances instead of plug-ins when you can. Avoid hairdryers and plug-in electric razors. Keep your distance from electrical appliances when in use. Do not sleep with electric blankets (however they can be used to warm up the bed and then turned off). Keep telephones, answering machines, and electric clocks away from your head while sleeping. Sit at least six feet away from your television.

✓ There are two kinds of radiation: ionizing and nonionizing. EMFs are nonionizing. In contrast, ionizing radiation (from atomic bombs, medical radiation treatments and X-rays) is much more harmful. Some ionizing radiation is unavoidable as it has contaminated our soil, water, and air. (A reverse osmosis water purifier can remove radioactive particles from drinking water.) We can, however, say no to unnecessary medical X-rays (most diagnostic X-rays are not medically necessary) and to airport-scanner searches.

✓ When, where and how much you sleep, as well as the quality of your sleep, have far-reaching biological consequences. The body has been programmed for millennia to sleep when it's dark and be awake during daylight. Our circadian rhythms govern our capacity for self-regulation and self-repair. It is best to go to sleep around 10:00 PM. To get good quality sleep, your room should be totally dark (including no LED lights from iPods, laptops, electronic readers, TV sets, alarm clocks, etc.) While sleep needs vary, most people need between seven to nine hours of mostly uninterrupted sleep per night. Using a cell phone just before going to bed increases the time it takes to get to sleep and reduces the quality of your sleep.

✓ Noise pollution disrupts sleep; it is also inflammatory and disrupts hormone balance and immunity.

CHAPTER 8

The Genetic Pathway

*Over time there is a greater and
greater chance that DNA damage will occur that
somehow escapes repair. . . . Such damage . . .
makes the cell less efficient. . . . This is the cause of
aging, according to many popular theories.*

—Gary L. Samuelson,
author of *The Science of Healing Revealed*

*Nutrition can alter the course of high-risk genes,
not only by turning these genes off but also
by inhibiting the resulting bad effects
produced by them.*

—Russell L. Blaylock, MD,
author of *Health and Nutrition Secrets*

I F, UP TO NOW, YOU HAVE THOUGHT that your longevity and how well you age is coded in your genes, you are not alone. However, this is a misconception. All life processes take place inside of cells, and DNA contains all the instructions necessary to set them in motion. What people frequently overlook is the fact that the DNA is not solely responsible for the fate of their cells. Different cellular environments give different instructions to genes. By changing the environment, you change how the genes function, and consequently, how you function. That's why the controlling factor is not the genes but the environment you create for them. What you eat, the toxins you are exposed to, and your thoughts can literally change the function of your genes. Ultimately, it is you, not the genes, who are in control.

Genes themselves are not set in stone. They are living structures, susceptible to damage, mutation, repair, and the instructions you give to them, depending on your living conditions. The closer your living environment—inside and outside of your body—is to that in which your genes originally evolved, the healthier and more stable your genes will be. Conversely, pervasive changes in the environment, such as we have been experiencing over the past century and a half, destabilize our genetic machinery. Nevertheless, there is much about your external and internal environment that you have control over, including your mindset, and these factors are powerful in determining how your genes express. For example if you have an abnormal BRCA gene (which increases the risk of breast cancer), it does not mean you will get breast cancer.

This is simply a possibility—unless you make it a reality with your thoughts, toxic exposures, diet, and lifestyle.

You Control Your Genes

Genes are a set of instructions that tell our bodies how to develop from a single cell into an entire human being. Only about one-quarter of our genes express (turn on) automatically, determining, for example, whether our eyes are blue or our hair is curly. Most genes merely offer thousands of possibilities—what *can* happen, not what *will* happen. Rather than thinking of genes as predetermined outcomes, think of them as a range of options—a set of "what-ifs." If certain circumstances are present, then specific genes will turn on and express in a particular way. If other circumstances are present, those same genes will express in a different way. Biochemist Roger Williams, author of *Nutrition Against Disease,* maintained that genes alone are entirely useless threads of chemicals. They do not determine our sickness or health. They act more like computer programs that sit dormant, essentially doing nothing, until you tell them what you want them to do. For something specific to happen, these genetic programs require an instruction, some sort of a trigger—environmental or psychological—in order for them to choose which option to express. You are in control of these triggers through your diet, lifestyle, and thoughts. You truly control your genes—including those that influence the aging process.

There isn't a single pharmaceutical that can up-regulate gene expression. Yet gene expression in well over 500 genes can be affected beneficially with simple changes in diet and lifestyle.

You Can Age Well with the Genes You Have

We often worry far more than we need to about genetic inheritance. Following the advent of human genome sequencing, scientists have redoubled their efforts to isolate the "aging gene." Numerous papers have been published holding out distant hope for "genetic therapies" for everything from wrinkles to heart disease. However, what you really need to know about aging is that you can age well with the genes you have. Are there genes that make you more susceptible to Alzheimer's and heart conditions? No doubt. Will these genes cause these diseases? No! Genes make the disease process possible, but they do not cause it. *To cause degeneration and disease, you have to turn off protective genes, activate disease-promoting genes, and then drive the disease process.* Consider that a century ago cancer affected only 3 percent of the American population. Now almost half of all Americans will develop cancer in their lifetime. Our genes haven't changed in the last century, but our diet, environment, and lifestyle have. It is not possible to blame our epidemic of degenerative diseases and premature aging on inherited genes. *The real problem is we are doing unprecedented damage to our genes, as well as giving them all the wrong instructions.*

Don't Mess with Your Genes

The most promising genetic therapy to postpone aging is to spare our genes the constant onslaught of nutritional deficiencies, toxins, stress, and radiation. The best part is that anyone can do this. Our daily living is reflected in the microenvironment we create for our cells. The environment in which our cells function is the single most important factor in how well we age. The environment is a trigger that causes genes to express in different ways, and you are creating that environment every moment of every day. You are constantly determining how your genes express with the foods you eat, the air you breathe, the water you drink, and the thoughts you think.

Tell Your Genes to Keep You Young

Unfortunately, in today's world, we are telling our genes to make us sick and age us prematurely. We are damaging our genes, giving them improper instructions, and in every way possible, causing them to malfunction. Through our nutritionally deficient diet, exposure to toxins, exposure to radiation, stress, lack of sleep, and other factors, not only are we instructing our genes to make us old and sick, but we are also shutting down the DNA repair genes that are there to protect us from premature aging and disease. We are doing everything just right to get old before our time.

To prevent or reverse premature aging, you have to:

Stop damaging your genes.
Support DNA repair.
Give your genes the correct instructions.

Gene Mutations Damage Your Health

Genes are crucial plans for creating, repairing, and reproducing an organism. Making random changes to the operating system will create chaos on your computer, and the same thing happens when you create random changes in genetic coding with mutations.

Mutations are unpredictable, permanent changes in genetic coding caused by malnutrition, toxins, and radiation.

Epigenetic Changes Give Wrong Instructions to Healthy Genes

Mutation changes the coding of genes and permanently alters their function. But there is another type of change that alters the function of genes *without* changing the coding itself, called epigenetic changes. *Epigenetic changes* result from environmental chemicals interacting with genes and interfering with their normal expression, and this is turning out to be a big problem. We normally test chemicals for safety by looking for genetic mutations. This type of testing is no longer adequate because we now know that environmental pollutants can cause aging and disease through epigenetic changes in the absence of actual mutations or structural damage to DNA. Worse, there is evidence that, like mutations, epigenetic changes can be passed on to future generations. This is one more reason to make the effort to avoid exposing yourself to environmental toxins and to do what is necessary to reduce your existing toxic load.

In addition to toxins, poor nutrition causes epigenetic changes. A mother's malnutrition, without changing the genes themselves, can permanently alter the expression of genes in her offspring. This is a major factor in the poor health of our current generation of children. Part of our cancer epidemic can be explained by our consumption of nutritionally deficient processed foods over several generations—even the nutritional deficiencies of your grandparents can show up in how your genes express and your susceptibility to disease. The toxins we are exposed to and what we eat have far-reaching consequences beyond the damage they do to ourselves and our own children. The entire future of the species is being affected.

Stop Damaging Your Genes

To protect yourself from DNA mutations, limit your exposure to the DNA-damaging toxins and radiation. As we age, our DNA repair capability is reduced, so as you grow older it becomes all the more important to protect your DNA from damage. Here are some things to look out for:

Ionizing radiation. About half the average person's exposure to ionizing radiation comes from diagnostic X-rays and medical radiation treatments. A number of researchers have estimated that up to 90 percent of X-rays have "little or no medical value," and are not medically justified. Decline all routine X-rays, and allow only those X-rays that are absolutely necessary. It is paradoxical that physicians, who put so much stock in the genetic origins of disease, are themselves inflicting massive genetic damage with toxic pharmaceuticals and radiation.

Nonionizing radiation. While not causing mutations, nonionizing radiation also has genetic repercussions. As a general rule, avoid close proximity or prolonged exposure to all types of electrical devices, electrical boxes, transformers, cell phones, cell phone towers, and high-voltage power lines.

Toxins. These include man-made industrial chemicals, prescription drugs, tobacco, and chemical residues in meat and dairy products such as hormones, PCBs and dioxins, fluoride, and metals such as mercury and lead. Foods heated to high temperatures or blackened (as in barbecuing) contain chemicals capable of causing gene mutations and cancer.

Support DNA Repair

Inherited genes are not causing our epidemic of premature aging and disease; it is damage to our genes that is causing these problems. Life in the twenty-first century is damaging our genes and creating mutations at an alarming rate. Fortunately, genetic damage can be repaired. Not only must we avoid damaging our genes in the first place, we also must provide our genes with the raw materials (nutrients) they need to repair themselves.

Genes get damaged all the time. This is normal, and it is why we have DNA repair systems. However, due to our poor diets and our massive exposure to toxins and radiation, our DNA repair systems are having a difficult time keeping up with all the damage. Critical DNA repairs are not getting done, and sometimes the genetic damage even disables the repair machinery itself.

If DNA is damaged and not repaired before the cell divides to form a new cell, the damage will become permanent and show up in all the new cells. The effects of this can range from minor to devastating, as the damage is cumulative. Damaged cells and genes can lead to premature aging and a variety of conditions, including fatigue, poor resistance to infections, psychological stress, social maladjustment, and cancer.

Certain nutrients are known to support the DNA repair process. You have to supply these nutrients or the repairs will not be made, and you will accumulate repair deficits, accelerate the aging process, and get sick. This is why nutritional deficiencies result in a similar kind of genetic damage as that caused by ionizing radiation. Critical nutrients include vitamins B_3, B_6, B_{12}, and folate, as well as zinc and L-carnitine. Most Americans are deficient in these nutrients. According to the USDA, 73 percent of Americans are deficient in zinc, 40 percent are deficient in B_{12}, and 80 percent are deficient in B_6. Augmenting your diet with high-quality supplements is essential.

Give Correct Instructions to Your Genes

When turned on, a single gene is capable of producing as many as 30,000 different proteins, each of which has a different role in the body and creates a different outcome. What determines which protein the gene will produce? The instructions it receives from its environment—and you create that environment. A lot of people think, for example, that genes cause cancer and that cancer runs in their families; therefore, they are going to get it. This is an old way of thinking, and it's a big mistake to think that way today. A study of twins, reported in a 2000 issue of the *New England Journal of Medicine*, concluded, "The overwhelming contributor to the causation of cancer in the populations of twins that we studied was the environment." A 2011 doctoral dissertation by John D. Clarke, a molecular and cellular biologist, proved that a diet rich in broccoli sprouts was able to prevent prostate cancer. Terry Wahls, MD, was able to reverse her multiple sclerosis without pharmaceuticals by eating a diet high in organic sulfur-rich foods, including broccoli. Again, the environment you create for your genes is far more important than the genes themselves in determining whether you get cancer, how long you are going to live, and what it would be like for you to get old.

For a moment, let's think about genes as computer programs; computer programs are designed to perform specific tasks such as word processing, e-mails, computer games, and so on. Within its intended area of function, each program is capable of doing a variety of different tasks, depending on what you ask it to do.

The chemical environment you create inside each cell determines what you ask your genes to do. You create those environments with your diet and lifestyle. Your level of physical activity, and the amount of sunlight, fresh air, and sleep you get, all influence the chemical environment produced in each cell. The pH inside your cells, the amount of sodium in your cells, the amount and kind of toxins in your cells, the hormones and hormone-like chemicals you have consumed, the electromagnetic environment you're exposed to, and your thoughts, beliefs, and emotions all create an environment that interacts with your unique set of genes to tell them what to do, resulting in how they express. One way or another, most of this is under your control.

Hormones are genetic switches, activating certain genes and deactivating certain others. It is extremely important to your health that you normalize hormone function. The correct hormone balance is anti-aging, and an imbalance will speed up the aging process. Hormone balance is why getting the right amount of sleep is so important and why stress hormones can kill you. One reason why sugar is such a dangerous toxin is that it unbalances your hormones. It is also why consuming meat and dairy products, and the hormones they contain, contributes to aging and disease.

Nutrients in your diet also interact with your genes. Scientists have discovered that vitamin D directly influences more than 200 genes. Included are genes connected to cancer and autoimmune diseases like multiple sclerosis. Running low on vitamin D at a critical juncture can and does mean the difference between a debilitating illness and excellent health. By the end of winter, more than half of all Americans are vitamin D deficient.

Studies of cancer patients have shown that lifestyle changes involving diet, exercise, and human interaction can alter the expression of hundreds of cancer-related genes in the direction of health. Meanwhile, stress hormones have been found to change gene expression for the worse. Further, stress hormones affect virtually every cell in the body, and the negative programming can remain even after the hormones have returned to their normal levels. The good news is that you can improve your health and reduce your biological age by influencing the expression of your genes through stress reduction and maintaining a positive outlook.

Ultimately what matters is not what genes you have but how they are expressed. You don't have control over which genes you inherited, but you do have control over how they express. Through your lifestyle choices, you tell your genes to turn on or off, which proteins to produce, and when to produce them. Genes run your life, but you run your genes—so ultimately you are in charge. Take care to give yourself the long, disease-free life you want.

The Bottom Line

- ✓ Despite popular belief, we control our genes; our genes do not control us. Genes respond to instructions we give them. Most genes are DNA codes that can be expressed in thousands of different ways, with thousands of different biological outcomes. We instruct our genes through the cellular environments we create with our lifestyle choices.

- ✓ For example, possessing the BRCA gene does not mean you will get breast cancer. Breast cancer is simply a possibility unless you make it a reality with your thoughts, toxic exposures, diet, and lifestyle.

- ✓ A healthy lifestyle includes a good diet, exercise, sunlight, fresh air, adequate sleep, systemic alkalinity, sodium-potassium balance, limiting toxic exposures, detoxification, hormonal balance, and a positive attitude that creates an optimal cellular environment for genetic expression supporting health and successful aging.

- ✓ Genes get damaged all the time. The damage can be repaired, and ideally repair keeps pace with damage. When it does not, mutations occur. Mutations introduce chaos into biological systems, leading to cancer and other types of disease. Epigenetic changes are another kind of damage to gene function but they do not alter the DNA code. These come from environmental chemicals and poor nutrition interacting with genes and interfering with their normal expression. Both mutated genes and epigenetic changes can be passed down through generations.

✓ Life in the twenty-first century is damaging our genes and creating mutations in unprecedented ways, and at an alarming rate. You can stop much of this damage by avoiding toxins as well as ionizing and nonionizing radiation wherever possible. See previous chapters for specifics.

✓ Support DNA repair by optimizing your nutrient intake, especially vitamins B_3, B_6, B_{12} and folate, zinc, and L-carnitine. Most Americans are deficient in one or more of these nutrients.

CHAPTER 9

The Medical Pathway

Doctors give drugs of which they know little,
into bodies, of which they know less, for diseases
of which they know nothing at all.

—Voltaire

Somewhere around 90 percent of surgery is a
waste of time, money, energy, and life.

—Dr. Robert Mendelsohn,
author of *Confessions of a Medical Heretic*

"THIS IS THE DARK AGE OF MEDICINE," said Henry Bieler, MD, in his book *Food Is Your Best Medicine.* Conventional medicine is a blunder of historic dimensions, and it is one of our leading causes of aging and disease. In the United States, medical

285

intervention is the leading cause of death. Astounding to say the least! How did that happen?

Where did we ever get the idea that we could help sick people by feeding them toxic chemicals or removing essential body parts? Yet this is the basis of conventional medicine. If you feed toxic chemicals to healthy people, you will make them sick. How then is it possible to give sick people toxic chemicals and make them well? People are not sick because they suffer from a drug deficiency or because they have body parts they don't need. Rather, they suffer from nutritional deficiencies and toxicities that disable their vital defense and repair mechanisms. Deficiency and toxicity are the two causes of all disease, and prescription drugs are toxins. These toxic drugs also create deficiencies. To keep ourselves young and in good repair, we need nutrients, not drugs. We also need a body with all of its organs in place and fully functioning.

The two cases where modern medicine does save lives are trauma care and crisis intervention. However, where aging and chronic illness are concerned, your first order of business is to protect yourself from the massive harm of conventional medicine, while mobilizing all the resources I have described so far in this book, to put yourself on the path of true wellness. The medical pathway is about replacing drugs and surgery with safe alternatives and shunning all unnecessary medical procedures, including any invasive screening, diagnostics, vaccinations, medical and dental X-rays, and much more. Consider that the price you may pay for conventional medicine's blunders is permanent damage to your health and quality of life, and perhaps life itself.

Please understand that the above in no way questions the good intentions and integrity of our physicians. Rather, it calls to your attention the unscientific body of knowledge they learned in school and the disastrous effects of applying that deeply flawed knowledge to real people. While some physicians have reached far beyond their training and are incorporating advanced science into their practices, they are still too few to have a major impact on the whole of medicine.

Looking at medical education in America, Sir George Pickering, MD, a professor of medicine at Oxford University and one of the twentieth century's most respected experts in medical education, said in a 1971 *British Medical Journal* article: "Medical education in the U.S. is, to a large extent, worship at the improbable shrine of worthless knowledge. We produce 'scientific illiterates' . . . who are not scientific in their approach to clinical questions or new technologies." Sadly, little has changed since he wrote that in 1971.

Vanessa's Story:
Hold the Zoloft, Pass the Broccoli

In her twenties, Vanessa was a promising young model. But at age forty-eight, she was already an old woman, ailing, tired, and spent. Thirty years earlier, Vanessa had been diagnosed with depression. Since then, she was a patient at some of the top medical centers in the country. She had been on numerous successive medications, none of which helped, and most of which made her even sicker. Vanessa's depression was

pronounced *untreatable*. In the meantime, her health problems multiplied. Her weight, cholesterol, and blood pressure
all went up, which prompted her doctors to prescribe more
drugs. When I met her, she was obese and suicidal, her skin
looked terrible, her hair was falling out, and she had no energy
at all. In the process of correcting her diet, I discovered that
Vanessa had a cerebral allergy to gluten. Once gluten-free,
Vanessa's thirty-year "untreatable" depression was cured in
forty-eight hours! Two years after she stopped taking prescription drugs, changed to a fresh plant-based diet, and got
on a good supplement program, Vanessa had fully recovered
from all her medical problems and had regained her youthful
energy and stunning beauty—looking fifteen years younger
than her chronological age.

Conventional Medicine Does
More Harm Than Good

Have you noticed that people on prescription drugs age faster?
Vanessa's case is tragically commonplace, and, in fact, she was
lucky to be able to reverse the aging and the damage done to her
body through routinely prescribed drugs. Drugs interfere with
the normal functioning of cells—which is why they are prescribed
in the first place. In the process of drug discovery, drug companies discard all compounds from which the body can easily rid
itself, selecting only those that bind to receptor sites inside the
cells and thus alter normal cell metabolism. In this way, modern

medicine attempts to control the outward symptoms of disease, without addressing its root causes: deficiency and toxicity. When this approach fails, the conventional response is to escalate the violence against your body, using surgery to remove the "misbehaving" parts. Like a protracted war, modern medical treatments disrupt and devastate the body, spreading the damage along every one of the Six Pathways:

Nutritional deficiencies. Antibiotics, anti-inflammatories, and steroids seriously damage the human digestive tract, impairing the ability to absorb nutrients. Diuretics strip nutrients, such as magnesium, calcium, potassium, zinc, and iodine. Cholesterol-lowering drugs cause CoQ_{10} deficiency, which can result in fatigue and congestive heart failure, as well as promote cancer. Chemotherapy drugs cause magnesium deficiency. Birth control pills lower vitamin C, folate, B_2, B_6, B_{12}, magnesium, and selenium. Hypertension drugs deplete vitamins C, B_1, B_6, and K, along with CoQ_{10}, calcium, magnesium, and zinc. Taking drugs for an extended period results in nutritional deficiencies that age your body and vastly increase your risk of every disease.

Toxic overload. All drugs are toxic to the body. Drugs disrupt normal cell chemistry, causing cells to malfunction, producing a variety of new diseases. To obscure the extent of the damage, the drug industry benignly refers to these new diseases as "side effects."

Psychological damage. Just being diagnosed with a serious illness is a shock from which some people are never able
to recover. When, on top of that, doctors estimate how long
a patient will live, or predict that he will never walk or see
again, they can so demoralize the patient as to create a self-
fulfilling prophecy.

Physical damage. Surgery, X-rays, radiation, and other
medical procedures physically damage the body, causing cellular malfunction and disease.

Genetic damage. Medical X-rays and certain drugs, such
as antidepressants, are known to cause genetic damage.
Genetic mutations can cause premature aging, cancer, and
other diseases, and the mutations may be passed on to future
generations.

Why You Shouldn't Always Trust Your Doctor

Don't get me wrong. I am not accusing doctors of being cyni-
cal and callous. Quite to the contrary, most go into their profession with a genuine desire to help people. But the education they
receive is, for the most part, hopelessly obsolete, unscientific, and
invalid—and the results are disastrous. Disease rates are soaring,
and the number of medical errors is alarming. Yet most people
trust their doctors.

Would you trust your new car to a mechanic who has been
trained to fix horse carriages? Of course not. Why then would you
trust your body to a physician who's been trained to "fix" you one

symptom at a time, in a system that has little basis in science? Let me explain what I mean.

Conventional Medicine Lags
Behind Current Science

Modern medicine dazzles the eye and intrigues the mind with an ever-growing array of sophisticated tools and cutting-edge technologies. It does do a first-rate job of treating medical emergencies. If you've been shot, been in a fire or a car accident, or suffered a heart attack, conventional medicine does a superb job. Your chances of survival are the highest today in all of recorded history. But when it comes to curing disease or promoting a lifetime of wellness, all this expensive medical technology is being misused and is woefully ineffective. In fact, most of conventional medicine's treatments for serious diseases, and especially for advanced cancer, are essentially worthless.

While appearing to be technologically advanced and claiming to be science-based, modern medicine long ago parted ways with modern science. Instead, it continues to rely on a seventeenth-century understanding of the human body. In 1687, Isaac Newton's discovery of the laws of motion gave rise to a mechanistic view of the universe and of the human body. Western-trained physicians began to treat the body as they would a clockwork mechanism, one part at a time, believing that they could control health simply by understanding the mechanics of the physical body.

In the early twentieth century, Albert Einstein challenged Newtonian physics and fundamentally changed the scientific view of the world. By proving that matter and energy are interchangeable, Einstein created a new paradigm for studying the laws of the universe—quantum physics—in which living organisms are regarded as networks of complex energy systems that interact with physical and cellular systems. We human beings are not Newtonian in nature, but rather Einsteinian. We are multidimensional energy systems, yet conventional medicine is stuck in its seventeenth-century view of the body as a mechanical clock with interchangeable parts. Because our bodies are complex energy systems, physicians in the future will be trained in physics rather than biology. No matter how many expensive gadgets it uses, conventional medicine is doomed to failure without the correct understanding of the true nature of the human body.

Most people believe that their doctor is using the latest science to treat them. Nothing could be further from the truth. Studies, including one by the U.S. Office of Technology Assessment, have concluded that *only 10 to 15 percent of conventional medical treatment has any basis in science*. It is in this small area, primarily crisis intervention and trauma care, that medicine excels. This means that 85 to 90 percent of medical practice has never been proven by scientific method to be safe and effective. The most recent study documenting this was published in the 2011 *Archives of Internal Medicine*. It found that even when doctors follow existing medical guidelines to the letter, 86 percent of the time they are using treatments that have little or no scientific support.

Doctors follow the existing guidelines, but there is no science behind the guidelines. In reality, the guidelines are based on the assumptions or opinions of the members of a guideline-drafting panel. Patients trust their doctors and the doctors trust the medical authorities, assuming that the professors who taught them and sit on the panels know what they are doing—but they don't. As a result, both doctors and patients underestimate the amount of harm that most drugs and surgeries do and overestimate the benefits. In fact, there is little or no evidence that many widely used treatments and procedures actually work better than various cheaper and safer alternatives, or even better than placebos.

Conventional medicine has been unable or unwilling to translate the enormous scientific advances of the last century into clinical practice. Our physicians get no training in scientifically advanced molecular medicine, which emphasizes cellular and molecular interventions with nontoxic nutrients. Because of their inadequate training, most physicians have no idea how to read, interpret, or understand scientific literature. In addition, most studies in the medical literature are poorly directed, deeply flawed, funded by organizations with vested interests, and often announce conclusions that are not supported by the data in the study. This is bad science, and it is why the eminent scientist Linus Pauling called most cancer research "a fraud."

Conventional medicine is now far behind current science, and the situation is so serious that the prestigious Institute of Medicine of the National Academy of Sciences studied the matter and issued a report in 2001. This shocking report, *Crossing the Quality Chasm*, concluded that, "Between the health care we now have and the health care we could have lies not just a gap but a chasm." The report also said: "The nation's health care delivery system has fallen short in its ability to translate knowledge into practice and to apply new technology safely and appropriately. . . . If the system cannot consistently deliver today's science and technology, it is even less prepared to respond to the extraordinary advances that surely will emerge during the coming decades."

The report concluded that conventional medical practice in America is so far off course at this point, there is no way it can be salvaged—it needs to be discarded and replaced with what the Academy called "a fundamental, sweeping redesign."

Conventional medicine waits for disease to happen. Then it attempts to suppress the symptoms with toxic drugs and invasive surgery, doing enormous, often irreparable—and sometimes even fatal—damage to the body. This irrational approach not only runs up the costs of health care but also leaves you sicker than when you started, makes your disease chronic, and may even kill you. This outmoded system needs to be replaced with science-based medicine. We must move away from the old focus on diagnosing and treating disease to a new paradigm of preventing disease and promoting wellness. We need to focus on creating health, longevity, and quality of life instead of managing disease with toxic drugs and surgery. The science to do so already exists, and the tide of popular opinion is slowly turning. Why, then, are our physicians still practicing "poison, slash, and burn" medicine that is ruining lives and bankrupting our country? Because there are formidable forces resisting the change.

Conventional Medicine Is a Business

Conventional medicine is an enormous industry whose survival is totally dependent on millions of people getting sick and staying sick. What would happen to all the hospitals, physician practices, drug companies, medical technology start-ups, and disease not-for-profits if they ever succeeded in preventing and curing chronic disease? Make no mistake, conventional medicine is big business, and the disease industry has little economic incentive to restore you to optimum health—*sick but not dead* is the financial sweet spot. That's why it is *your* job to take care of your own health, and I urge you to take it seriously.

An average cost of hip replacement in America is about $40,000. Coronary bypass surgery: $65,000. A one-year supply of Enbrel, a commonly prescribed rheumatoid arthritis drug: up to $25,000. Three out of four health care dollars (or roughly $2 trillion out of the $2.7 trillion total cost of U.S. health care) are spent treating entirely preventable chronic conditions. It costs a lot more to fix something after it is broken than to prevent it from breaking in the first place. Yet conventional medicine makes almost no attempt to prevent disease. It also does an extremely poor job in treating chronic disease, and physicians appear to be oblivious to the fact that their treatments do more harm than good.

Conventional Medicine Is a Cult

Have you asked your doctor's advice on nutrition or alternative care? Chances are their advice only directed you back to drugs or surgery. Despite the wealth of scientific evidence to the contrary, conventional medicine remains curiously entrenched in its methods. Part of the problem is that at no time during their education or career are conventional doctors encouraged to question existing practices. In fact, the opposite is true. Physicians can lose their license by failing to adhere to "prevailing standards of practice." Medical authorities can revoke a license even if no patient has been harmed, no patient has complained, or if the condition of the patients has actually improved. In other words, even if your doctors know of a safe, alternative treatment, *it is not safe for them to give it to you.* This makes change very difficult, and it is one reason why medicine has fallen so far behind our rapidly advancing science.

Conventional Medicine Is a Perfect Crime

From medical errors to adverse drug reactions to unnecessary procedures, conventional medicine is literally killing us, and the numbers are right there in the medical statistics. A number of analyses, including those in Dr. Carolyn Dean's 2005 book, *Death by Modern Medicine*; Gary Null's 2010 book, *Death by Medicine*; the 1991 *Harvard Medical Practice Study*; the 1994 *Journal of the American Medical Association* article "Error in Medicine," and others have shown that conventional medicine has caused more harm than good. The authors of these analyses took statistics right from the most respected medical and scientific journals and investigative reports by the Institute of Medicine. They have clearly demonstrated that medical intervention is the leading cause of death in America, killing about 1 million people per year. According to the

2011 *Health-Grades Hospital Quality and Clinical Excellence Study,*
the incidence rate of medical harm is now more than 40,000 each
day. The 2003 "Death by Medicine" report issued by the Nutrition
Institute of America concluded: "Our estimated ten-year total of
7.8 million iatrogenic [doctor-induced] deaths is more than all
the casualties from all the wars fought by the U.S. throughout its
entire history."

It is significant to note that while conventional medicine kills
about a million Americans per year and injures tens of millions, the
medical establishment, the drug industry, and government regula-
tors attempt to ban and restrict the use of vitamins and herbs that
kill no one. Why isn't conventional medicine held responsible for all
these deaths? Because it has made them so commonplace, they are
accepted as normal. A combination of powerful business interests
and relentless brainwashing throughout the medical establishment
and mass media has created a culture where convention prevails
over science and common sense. How many people religiously get
their annual flu shots and their mammograms? Yet both of these,
along with hundreds of other routine medical procedures, have
been shown to be of limited value and, potentially, of considerable harm.

Screening Doesn't Prevent Anything

The only way to prevent disease is to supply your cells with the
nutrients they need and protect them from toxins and physical
harm, which includes most "preventive" medical care. The medical establishment aggressively promotes screening for cancer and

other diseases. But the kind of screening they do does not *prevent* anything. What it does is offer you a trade-off between a potential risk of a late diagnosis (in case you do eventually get the disease you are being screened for) and a very real and tangible risk of harm from the test itself.

Colonoscopy

Since Katie Couric's televised colonoscopy in March 2000, colorectal cancer screening rates have soared. Colorectal cancer is the second-leading cause of cancer-related deaths and the third-most-commonly diagnosed cancer in the United States. The American Cancer Society recommends that, starting at age fifty, everyone get a colonoscopy every ten years, or a CT colonography (virtual colonoscopy) every five years. According to the Centers for Disease Control, 59 percent of the U.S. population between ages fifty and seventy-five follow these guidelines. Upon turning fifty, people line up in droves for the dreaded colonoscopies, hoping to catch this deadly cancer before it claims their lives. Yet there are simple dietary steps everyone can take to virtually eliminate the risk of getting colon cancer. Recall from Chapter 3, "The Nutrition Pathway," that never browning your meat brings down your odds of getting colon cancer, and consuming mostly whole plant-based foods brings the risk of any cancer close to zero. On the other hand, a colonoscopy has a number of well-known risks and side effects, among them: disruption of intestinal flora, colon perforation, post-operative delayed bleeding, infection, increased risk of deferred strokes, heart attacks, pulmonary embolisms, and false negatives.

Virtual colonoscopy adds to the risk. According to the American College of Gastroenterology, virtual colonoscopies miss 27 percent of colorectal lesions, including precancerous colon polyps and actual cancerous tumors. When virtual colonoscopy does find a problem, to treat it, you'll need to undergo a regular colonoscopy anyway. False positive readings are also common. Plus, abdominal CT scans expose you to a massive dose of radiation.

Bottom line: Unless you are suspected of already having colon cancer, colonoscopies, both actual and virtual, are dangerous medical procedures that expose you to physical harm, toxic drugs, and disruption of vital processes in the body, while doing nothing to lower your risk of colon cancer. If you are serious about preventing colon cancer and staying biologically young, change your diet and stay away from CT scanners and other unnecessary medical tests.

Diagnostic X-Rays

Americans today are exposed to seven times more radiation from diagnostic X-rays than they were in 1980. Most of the average person's lifetime radiation exposure comes from diagnostic X-rays, yet there is no medical justification for as much as 90 percent of them, including routine X-rays like mammograms. Mammograms expose your body to radiation that can be hundreds of times greater than a chest X-ray. Mammograms not only increase the risk of developing breast cancer, they also increase the risk of it spreading. Regarding mammograms, a 1995 study in the *Lancet* concluded, "The benefit is marginal, the harm caused is substantial, and the costs incurred are enormous." Each additional radiation exposure, no matter how small, increases the risk of cancer. This is why you should refuse all but the most necessary medical X-rays.

X-rays cause cancer. This is why radiologists and technicians who are around X-ray equipment every day have more cancer than the general population. John Gofman, MD, PhD, was both a medical doctor and a nuclear physicist. He was one of the world's leading experts on radiation damage, and his groundbreaking book, *Radiation from Medical Procedures in the Pathogenesis of Cancer and Ischemic Heart Disease,* was published in 1999. Gofman's three decades of research into the effects of low-dose radiation on humans indicated that medical X-rays play an essential role in about 75 percent of all breast cancers. Cancer statistics show that breast cancer has increased since the introduction of mammographic screening in 1983. In fact, one form of breast cancer, ductal carcinoma *in situ*, has increased more than 300 percent. A 2008 study in the *Archives of Internal Medicine* found the start of mammography screening programs throughout Europe was associated with an increased incidence of breast cancer.

In addition to radiation damage we have already discussed, there are other reasons not to do routine mammograms. Mammography compresses the breasts (often painfully), which could cause any existing malignant cells to spread. Mammograms have a high rate of false positives. About 5 percent of mammograms suggest further testing; more than 90 percent of those are false positives. This results in unnecessary expense, emotional trauma, needless biopsies, and other unnecessary surgical procedures.

Mammograms also produce a high rate of false negatives; a false negative could cost you your life. According to the National Cancer Institute, for women in the forty to forty-nine age group, the rate of missed tumors is 40 percent. The truth is mammograms don't save lives. Research shows that adding an annual mammogram to a careful physical examination of the breasts does not improve breast cancer survival rates.

Fortunately, there is a better option. In addition to physical examination, physicians practicing advanced medicine use a safe, accurate, and inexpensive diagnostic test called a thermogram. Thermography measures the temperature of the breast, and there is no need for any mechanical pressure or ionizing radiation. Best of all, this technique is so sensitive, it can detect breast cancer as much as a decade earlier than a mammogram. The increased blood flow to a growing tumor makes that area warmer than the surrounding tissue. This temperature differential can be accurately measured, with no false negatives and few false positives, without any danger or discomfort to the patient.

CT Scans

Another serious problem is the widespread use of CT (computed tomography) scans, originally known as computed axial tomography (CAT) scans. The use of these X-ray scanners has increased dramatically over the last two decades. More than 75 million scans are now being performed in the United States annually. CT scans can image the entire human body within seconds, producing high-definition images that provide physicians with an incredibly detailed view of the organs and tissues deep within us.

While CT scans can be beneficial in certain situations, like serious injury from multiple traumas, routine overuse of these devices is exposing patients to an enormous amount of unnecessary radiation. Two studies published in the *Archives of Internal Medicine* in 2009 show that healthy people are being exposed to excessive, cancer-causing radiation for clinically dubious screening purposes.

Recall that there is no known "safe" dose of radiation. In light of this reality, consider that a single CT coronary artery angiogram can deliver the same amount of radiation as 310 chest X-rays. The studies mentioned above found enormous variations in the amount of radiation being delivered by different CT imaging facilities. The difference between the highest and lowest doses for the same type of scan was thirteenfold! Some people have received grossly excessive radiation during their scans, to the point that their hair began falling out. The researchers estimated that the CT scans done in 2007 alone will result in approximately 29,000 future cases of cancer, and this estimate is most likely conservative. Anyone with a nutritional deficiency or a poorly functioning DNA repair system will be especially vulnerable to radiation damage.

Biopsy

Even a needle biopsy is dangerous. Needle biopsies are routinely used for diagnosing cancer. But they are not safe! As early as 1940, medical experts warned that needle biopsies could cause cancer cells to break away from a tumor and spread to other parts of the body. A 2007 study in the *British Medical Journal* indicates that biopsies do exactly that—spread the cancer. If you have a needle biopsy, you are 50 percent more likely to have your cancer spread. The body is smart enough to build a protective wall around tumors to prevent metastasis. Then we are dumb enough to poke a hole in this protective capsule, allowing cancer cells to spill directly into the bloodstream or lymphatic system and spread throughout the body.

Prescription Drugs Create Disease

"One of the first duties of the physician is to educate the masses not to take medicine," said Canadian physician Sir William Osler, who has been called the "father of modern medicine." One of the more tragic aspects of conventional medicine is the use of toxic chemicals called prescription drugs. Everyone wants a magic pill to cure disease, but there is no such thing. All drugs do is suppress symptoms, while the risk of taking them far exceeds potential benefits. Prescription drugs are one of the leading causes of disease as well as the third-leading cause of death in the United States. Drugs are major contributors to our aging epidemic.

Taking any drug disrupts your normal body chemistry. Prescription drugs create both deficiency and toxicity, damaging immunity and reducing the body's overall resistance to disease. This is why properly prescribed prescription drugs hospitalize more than 2 million and kill an estimated 450,000 (officially 100,000) people every year. Side effects and drug interactions decrease the quality of life for tens of millions more. By the time you are on five prescriptions, serious repercussions are unavoidable. Yet 46 percent of Medicare patients take five or more prescription drugs. These hapless patients are the victims of professional malpractice.

Americans Are Overmedicated

According to the U.S. Centers for Disease Control and Prevention, almost half of all Americans take at least one prescription drug, and more than 20 percent take three or more. Our doctors write roughly 3 billion prescriptions per year, and the numbers are growing. Americans are bombarded with TV ads to ask their doctors for prescription drugs. As a result, we consume more prescription drugs per person than any other country. This helps to explain why we are in such poor health and why our health care system is one of the worst-performing in the world.

We use drugs as a Band-Aid to get rid of symptoms and conditions that should be addressed with proper diet, exercise, lifestyle, diaphragm breathing, water intake, sleep, fasting/detoxification, and prayer/meditation/stillness as our first line of defense. "We are taking way too many drugs for dubious or exaggerated ailments," says Dr. Marcia Angell, former editor of the *New England Journal of Medicine* and author of *The Truth About the Drug Companies.* "What the drug companies are doing now is promoting drugs for long-term use to essentially healthy people. Why? Because it's the biggest market." Today doctors prescribe antidepressants even in the absence of serious symptoms, just because the patient is going through a divorce, for example, while potent drugs like beta-blockers are being pushed as a "prophylactic measure."

Almost No One Needs Long-Term Medication

Some people are alarmed at the thought of not taking their drugs. They think that they need their drugs to lower their blood pressure, treat their depression, or control their diabetes. In truth, virtually no one needs a drug. It is difficult to think of a prescription drug for which there is not an alternative treatment that is safer, less expensive, and more effective. Every time independent researchers take a serious look at a prescription drug, they find it to be dangerous—so why take them? Find an alternative doctor who will help you get well, not make you a lifelong customer of the pharmaceutical companies, the insurance companies, and the medical establishment.

Remember, no drug, no matter how common, is ever safe. When it comes to modern industrial medicine, there is no safety in numbers. In fact, quite the opposite is true. By widely promoting dangerous disease-causing drugs, the industry lowers our expectations of safety and efficacy and hides long-term effects of these drugs. Let's have a look at some of the most common medications and the harm they do.

Cholesterol Drugs

High cholesterol is not the cause of heart disease; inflammation is. Inflammation oxidizes cholesterol. Whether your cholesterol is high or low doesn't matter. Oxidized cholesterol is the problem. The solution is to prevent inflammation, not lower cholesterol. Pfizer's Lipitor is the bestselling drug of all time. Up to 80 million

Americans have elevated cholesterol, and millions are being prescribed statin drugs to lower their cholesterol. Half of all men and
a third of all women ages sixty-five to seventy-four are on statins.
Statin drugs do lower cholesterol, but that doesn't do you much
good, and the toxic side effects are horrendous.

The body uses cholesterol to make repairs. Cholesterol doesn't
cause heart disease any more than the Red Cross causes disasters.
So lowering cholesterol with drugs to prevent heart attacks makes
no sense at all. Medical statistics clearly show that statins have
failed to reduce heart attacks or overall mortality. In fact, statins
are known to *cause* congestive heart failure, and there has been
a frightening increase since the introduction of statins. In Crete,
the home of the healthy Mediterranean diet, there are virtually
no heart attacks despite average cholesterol levels well over 200.
There are as many heart attacks in people with cholesterol levels
under 200 as those whose levels are over 300, and half of all heart
attacks occur in people with perfectly normal cholesterol levels.
The French have the highest average cholesterol in Europe, around
250, but the lowest incidence of heart disease and half the heart
attacks we have in the United States.

Despite the fact that cholesterol drugs provide no health benefits, physicians continue to enthusiastically prescribe them.
Meanwhile,the harm they do is mounting daily.

Here is a list of conditions that have been linked to statins:

ALS	hepatitis	neuropathies
Alzheimer's	high blood sugar	pancreatitis
amnesia	homicidal impulses	Parkinson's disease
anxiety	hostility	plantar fasciitis
cancer	impaired memory	respiratory problems
cataracts	impotence	sexual dysfunction
confusion	insomnia	sleep disorders
depression	joint pain	stomach ulcers
disorientation	kidney failure	stroke
dizziness	liver damage	tremors
dry "crocodile" skin	loss of libido	urinary problems
heart failure	muscle pain and weakness	vertigo

Many side effects don't occur until weeks and sometimes years after commencing the drug. Cancer is one long-term side effect that may be missed, because most human studies with statins are time-limited. In studies with rodents, statins have caused cancer in every study, and in one human study reported in a 1996 issue of the *New England Journal of Medicine,* breast cancer rates went up 1,500 percent among statin users.

Cholesterol is best controlled by eating a good diet, getting sugar out of your life, supplementing with essential fatty acids, and exercising regularly. Take supplements with antioxidants like vitamins C and E, and omega-3 fatty acids, which are far more effective than statins in reducing both heart disease and all-cause mortality.

Birth Control Pills

Birth control pills seriously disrupt your body's hormonal balance and cause every kind of disease from depression to cancer. A 1991 study in the *Journal of the National Cancer Institute* found that women who take birth control pills for five years or more increase their risk of getting liver cancer by 550 percent over those who have never taken them. Birth control pills upset the ecology of the gut, leading to problems with digestion, nutrient absorption, the production of toxins, immune suppression, and accelerated aging.

TNF Blockers

Tumor necrosis factor (TNF) blockers are used to treat inflammatory and autoimmune diseases such as Crohn's disease and rheumatoid arthritis. The FDA has ordered makers of these drugs to include a "black box warning" about an increased risk of cancer in children and adolescents. This is the most severe warning that the FDA can place on a product without withdrawing it from the market. The FDA was forced into this action after numerous reports of children developing cancer while taking these drugs. The FDA analyzed the reports and concluded, in its *Ongoing Safety Review of*

Tumor Necrosis Factor (TNF) Blockers (August 4, 2009), that "there is an increased risk of lymphoma and other cancers associated with the use of these drugs in children and adolescents." It would be foolhardy to think they are not risky for adults as well. In addition, TNF blockers are known immunosuppressants. They lower your ability to fight infections. None of this is good for your longevity.

Antibiotics

Most people think of antibiotics as one of the greatest triumphs of conventional medicine. They are not! *Antibiotics are one of conventional medicine's greatest blunders.* Antibiotics are deadly toxins. Their purpose is to treat infections by killing bacteria. But here is the problem: they also destroy beneficial bacteria upon which your health and life depend. Gut bacteria play vital roles in many body functions, including digestion and immunity. Seventy percent of your immune system is located in the intestines, and its proper functioning depends on the proper assortment of beneficial bacteria in the gut. These bacteria also degrade toxins, produce essential vitamins and fats, and help with nutrient absorption. Astonishingly, there are more bacteria living in your intestines than you have cells in your body (bacteria are much smaller than human cells). In a way, they are comparable to an essential body organ, like the liver or lungs. *Antibiotics cripple this organ—permanently!*

Taking an antibiotic, even once in a lifetime, can leave you permanently damaged, causing a cascade of problems, including impaired immunity, gastrointestinal diseases, obesity, allergies, autoimmune diseases, diabetes, cancer, heart disease, mental and behavioral disorders, and accelerated aging. The more times you take antibiotics and the longer you take them, the worse it gets. The assortment of bacteria in your gut is unique to you. By indiscriminately killing all bacteria, antibiotics permanently alter your intestinal flora. Once destroyed, it is at least extremely difficult, and probably impossible, to restore your unique population back to normal. This can leave you with lasting weakness where there was once strength.

Stripping your gut of its natural balance of healthy bacteria promotes an overgrowth of harmful microorganisms, including parasites, mycoplasma, fungi, yeasts like Candida, and hostile bacteria such as Pseudomonas, Clostridium, and Klebsiella. This problem is called *dysbiosis*. Dysbiosis is dangerous because these harmful microorganisms produce many toxins, and these toxins can cause dysfunction of the endocrine glands, resulting in hypothyroidism and adrenal insufficiency, as well as numerous cognitive and neurological problems similar to multiple sclerosis and amyotrophic lateral sclerosis. Research published online in the 2012 *FASEB Journal* also suggests that dysbiosis can cause heart attacks, and, conversely, that maintaining healthy intestinal flora may help reduce heart attack risk. The study's author, John E. Baker, PhD, from the Division of Cardiothoracic Surgery at the Medical College of Wisconsin in Milwaukee, says the study's discovery of "the biochemical link between intestinal bacteria, their metabolites, and injury to the heart will reduce the risk of death from a heart attack and, coupled with the use of probiotics, will ultimately be able to improve the overall cardiovascular health of the human population." Gerald Weissmann, MD, editor-in-chief of the *FASEB*

Journal, said, "We may soon evaluate our body's susceptibility to disease by looking at the microbes that inhabit the gut."

Good health begins in the intestinal tract. With the exception of oxygen, all nutrition enters the body through the intestines. If food is not properly broken down, it will ferment and putrefy in the gut, producing powerful toxins that poison you. Once food is properly digested, nutrients from the food must be absorbed through the intestinal walls into the bloodstream. Good bacteria facilitate this absorption, while the damage done to gut tissue by harmful flora impedes it. Thus, destruction of helpful bacteria results in deficiency and toxicity—the two causes of all disease.

Food allergies, immunodeficiency syndromes, and a variety of intestinal disorders result from altered flora. Damage done by antibiotics has led to an epidemic of digestive problems, and the proof is the astounding quantity of over-the-counter digestive aids sold every year. Sadly, most doctors are still unaware that the antibiotics they prescribed have caused their patients' digestive problems.

More and more studies are showing a relationship between the use of antibiotics and cancer. A 2004 study in the *Journal of the American Medical Association* determined that women who have taken antibiotics are at increased risk for developing breast cancer, and *as the number of prescriptions for antibiotics increases, the risk of breast cancer steadily climbs.* The researchers suggested that antibiotics kill off bacteria needed to metabolize and remove estrogen in the gut. This causes an estrogen excess that stimulates the growth of cancer. Compared to women who took no antibiotics, those who had taken fewer than twenty-five antibiotic prescriptions had a 50 percent greater risk of breast cancer, while those who had taken more than twenty-five prescriptions had a 200 percent greater risk.

Widespread use of antibiotics creates antibiotic-resistant bacteria. These bacteria are now ravaging our hospitals and moving out into the general population. They cause illnesses that are difficult, if not impossible, to treat with antibiotics.

Taking an antibiotic even once in your lifetime can start a chain of events that will devastate your health. Taking antibiotics often, or for long periods, is virtually certain to cause lifelong health problems. Fortunately, *there is no need for antibiotics.* Antibiotics address only the symptoms of disease—the infection. Meanwhile, the real problem—the reason your immune system is depressed— is ignored. There are much safer, more effective, natural ways to deal with infections. Best of all is to prevent them with immune-enhancing nutrients such as vitamins A, C, D, E, and zinc. Natural antibiotics like wild oregano and olive leaf extract can be used to treat infections. Doctors and hospitals can use intravenous vitamin C or oxygen, electromagnetic, and ultraviolet light therapies for serious infections. The problem is most physicians are so far behind the science, they are not even aware of these therapies.

A properly functioning intestinal tract is one of your first lines of defense against disease. Conversely, an improper assortment of flora and declining levels of friendly intestinal bacteria precipitate the onset of chronic disease. Antibiotics contribute to virtually every imaginable disease from the common cold to autism to psoriasis. Also important to note, dysbiosis is a major contributor to our leading diseases of aging: cancer, cardiovascular diseases, and neurodegenerative diseases. *Dysbiosis impairs the body's repair function, causing degenerative disease and accelerating the aging process.* To help yourself, avoid antibiotics and supplement with high-quality probiotics. A good idea is to include raw, live-culture sauerkraut or kimchi in your diet.

Vaccines

Another colossal blunder enshrined by conventional medicine is vaccinations. The purpose of vaccinations is to prevent infectious disease. The problem is there is no scientific evidence that immunizations prevent disease. No vaccine has ever been scientifically proven in double-blind, placebo-controlled studies to be safe or effective. Meanwhile, the existing evidence indicates they are not safe and are only marginally effective, if at all.

The dramatic decline of infectious diseases, such as smallpox, diphtheria, and polio, is often cited as proof of vaccinations' effectiveness. The truth is the incidence of infectious disease declined before the introduction of vaccines—in other words, vaccines get credit for something they did not do. This decline is due to numerous factors, including lack of famine, better sanitation, safe water supplies, good sewage systems, less crowded living conditions, and herd immunity. For example, in 1950, the polio epidemic was at its height in Great Britain. By the time the polio vaccine was introduced in 1956, polio had already declined by 82 percent. In the United States, scarlet fever, cholera, typhoid, plague, and yellow fever all disappeared without vaccinations, and when outbreaks of measles and rubella do occur, more than 90 percent of the cases are in vaccinated children.

Regarding the common flu shot, numerous studies have found flu shots to be essentially worthless. Consider this study published in the *Lancet:* Absenteeism of more than 100,000 employees was noted each winter for three years and the conclusion was that flu shots did not confer *any* protection. Likewise, here is what a 2012 report on influenza vaccines from the Center for Infectious Disease Research and Policy at the University of Minnesota had to say:

"Applying rigorous scientific methodology to this issue clearly shows that current influenza vaccines do not offer the level of protection necessary to significantly lessen influenza morbidity and mortality. In fact, despite significant increases in influenza vaccine coverage for those over 65 years of age since the late 1990s, a minimal impact on influenza morbidity and mortality has been noted in this country."

In plain English, flu shots don't work. Even worse, they damage your health.

Here is what Australian researcher Viera Scheibner, PhD, had to say in her book *Vaccination* after investigating some 60,000 pages of medical literature on vaccination: "Immunizations, including those practiced on babies, not only did not prevent any infectious diseases; they caused more suffering and more deaths than has any other human activity in the entire history of medical intervention." Canadian physician Dr. Guylaine Lanctot, author of the bestseller *The Medical Mafia,* put it this way: "The medical authorities keep lying. Vaccination has been an assault on the immune system.

It actually causes a lot of illnesses. We are actually changing our genetic code through vaccination. . . . 100 years from now we will know that the biggest crime against humanity was vaccines." Renowned pediatrician and author Dr. Robert Mendelsohn was equally direct in his book *Confessions of a Medical Heretic*: "Much of what you have been led to believe about immunization simply isn't true. If I were to follow my deeper convictions, I would urge you to reject all inoculations for your child. . . . There is no convincing scientific evidence that mass inoculations can be credited with eliminating any childhood disease."

Professor George Vithoulkas, an international authority on homeopathic medicine, said this in his 1996 acceptance speech to the Swedish Parliament at the presentation of the Right Livelihood Awards (sometimes referred to as the "Alternative Nobel Prize"): "These chronic diseases, including hay fever, asthma, cancer, and AIDS, are the result of wrong interventions upon the organism by conventional medicine. . . . The immune systems of the Western population, through strong chemical drugs and repeated vaccinations, have broken down. . . . Medicine, instead of curing diseases, is actually the cause of the degeneration of the human race."

Vaccinations damage immunity and inflame the brain. When multiple vaccinations are given within a short period, this can cause chronic brain inflammation resulting in the learning and behavioral problems that we see in our young and the Alzheimer's and Parkinson's we see in our elderly.

Vaccines contain highly toxic mercury compounds, formaldehyde, and aluminum. Aluminum has been added to vaccines for about ninety years in the belief it spurs the body to produce disease-fighting antibodies. Eighteen of the thirty-six vaccines children get contain large doses of aluminum, up to forty-six times the maximum dose considered safe by the regulatory agencies. Pneumonia, tetanus, and HPV shots all contain aluminum, adding to the lifetime accumulation of aluminum in adults. Research has demonstrated that aluminum is an accumulative neurotoxin. It has a tendency to concentrate in the hippocampus, an area of the brain vital to crucial functions, including learning, memory, and behavior, causing neurological disorders in children and adults.

As we age, our brain becomes progressively more inflamed, and aluminum accelerates and magnifies that inflammation. Aluminum causes a number of diseases by displacing iron from its protective proteins, raising the level of free iron in the body. This triggers intense inflammation, free radical generation, and lipid peroxidation, damaging genes and tissues and accelerating the aging process. There is also powerful evidence that aluminum worsens the effects of other toxins, such as pesticides, herbicides, mercury, and fluoride. In essence, accumulating aluminum is making your brain age faster. The incidence of neurological disorders like Alzheimer's, ALS, Parkinson's, and multiple sclerosis is exploding because we are bioaccumulating toxins, like aluminum from vaccines, at an unprecedented rate.

Vaccines also contain viruses, and certain viruses have been associated with cancer. For example, a monkey virus, SV40, found in polio vaccine, has been proven to cause cancer and to be responsible for an outbreak of lung, brain, bone, and lymphatic cancers in those who received the polio vaccine decades ago. Two 2002 studies in the *Lancet* estimated that up to half of the 55,000 annual cases of non-Hodgkin's lymphoma can be attributed to polio vaccine received decades ago. A growing number of researchers are now attributing the epidemics of leukemia, asthma, autoimmune disease, cerebral palsy, infantile convulsions, sudden infant death syndrome, and childhood cancer to vaccinations.

Vaccinations have never been proven effective. On the contrary, they damage your health and accelerate the aging process—avoid them.

Ninety Percent of Surgeries Are Unnecessary

Surgery works very well to correct physical problems, such as birth defects and injuries from accidents or sports. However, surgery does not solve disease problems. Unfortunately, most surgery in the United States is performed to address systemic diseases like heart disease and cancer, wasting resources and harming the patient. These diseases are the result of cellular malfunction, and the proper way to treat them is to restore normal function to the cells with good nutrition and detoxification. Surgery is dangerous and damaging to the body, and it should never be performed unless there is absolutely no alternative. There is almost always an alternative. Even minor surgery unleashes a flood of free radicals, causing inflammation throughout the body, and suppressing the immune system.

More unnecessary surgery is being done today than ever before. Dr. Robert Mendelsohn, in *Confessions of a Medical Heretic,* estimated that around 90 percent of surgery is "a waste." He cites one independent review of people recommended for surgery in which most of the patients did not need surgery and half of them needed no medical treatment at all. In another case, a hospital oversight committee reviewed surgically removed tissues to find that most tissues being removed were healthy. In the year prior to the formation of the committee, the hospital performed 262 appendectomies. After the committee was formed, that number dropped to sixty-two. In March 1997, the Physicians Committee for Responsible Medicine published a statement saying that only 10 percent of hysterectomies are justified. In addition to rarely being necessary, surgery is risky. The possibilities of surgical error or complications from anesthesia and infection are very real, while the physical, mental, and emotional shocks to the body accelerate the aging process.

Surgery Increases Inflammation

Surgery is a traumatic assault on the body, causing a substantial increase in the production of inflammatory chemicals. Inflammation damages genes and tissues, causing telomere shortening, premature aging, and lower resistance to disease. High levels of inflammation have been shown to increase cancer cell adhesion and to stimulate the production of new blood vessels that feed tumors.

Heart Bypass

A heart bypass operation is a prime example of unnecessary surgery. In 1992, Nortin Hadler, MD, a professor of medicine at the University of North Carolina Medical School, concluded that 95 to 97 percent of the coronary bypass surgeries done that year were unnecessary—even though patients are usually told that without the surgery they will die. In truth, virtually all coronary disease is preventable with diet, supplements, and exercise. Likewise, coronary disease is reversible, as pioneers like Nathan Pritikin, Dr. Dean Ornish, and others have proven.

Hip Implants Poison Your Cells

About 250,000 Americans over fifty undergo hip replacement surgery each year, unknowingly exposing themselves to dangerous levels of toxic metals. A 2012 study in the *British Medical Journal (BMJ)* found toxic cobalt and chromium ions in the tissues of patients with all-metal hip implants. Cobalt-chromium implants have been known to release metal ions into the local tissue, damaging bones and muscles and causing long-term disability in some patients. Studies have also shown that the metal ions can spread through the bloodstream, into the major organs, and damage chromosomes causing heart disease and, potentially, cancer.

In May 2011, after Johnson & Johnson recalled the Articular Surface Replacement, the U.S. Food and Drug Administration ordered the makers of all-metal replacements to study how frequently they fail. In February 2012, Dr. Mathias Bostrom, an orthopedic surgeon at the Hospital for Special Surgery in New York City, reported in an interview with *USA Today* that tens of thousands of patients with faulty replacements might have lasting, debilitating damage. Michael Carome, deputy director of Public Citizen's Health Research Group, in a release issued with the *BMJ*'s findings, said, "This is one very large uncontrolled experiment exposing millions of patients to an unknown risk. We will only find out about the safety of these devices after large numbers of people have already been exposed." A good rule is to never put things in the body that are not natural to the body.

Your hips, just like the rest of your body, are self-repairing, living organisms. When properly maintained, they will last a lifetime. Preventive maintenance starts with a good diet. Follow the guidelines in this book. Do not consume the Big Four, and do eat a diet rich in organic, fresh, whole plant foods. Do not eat processed foods. Lose excess weight. Supplements such as vitamin C, quercetin, glucosamine, and chondroitin help to prevent damage to the hip joint. Regular workouts, for at least twenty minutes a day, will help to keep the muscles that support the hips and legs strong. Walking, dancing, biking, tennis, or swimming are all good choices. They will help stabilize the hip joints. If your doctor recommends hip replacement surgery, consider other options first, such as rebuilding the hip joint with a good diet and detoxification. There are lots of alternative practitioners who help people avoid surgery.

Eye Surgery

The most frequent surgical procedure in people older than sixty-five is cataract surgery, costing Medicare alone more than $3.5

billion per year and rising. By age eighty, half of all Americans have cataracts. Yet gradual loss of vision is not part of the normal aging process. It is a disease process. Cataract surgery, like most other elective surgery, is unnecessary.

Cataracts are a clouding of the eye's natural lens. They are caused by free radical oxidative damage, and high-sugar diets are known to be a contributing factor. Cataracts can be prevented with a good diet and antioxidant supplementation. A diet high in fresh spinach, kale, and broccoli is known to dramatically reduce the risk of cataracts. Supplementing with carotenes, zinc, and vitamins B_1, B_2, C, D, and E have been proven enormously protective. Combining a good diet with these supplements will make you virtually cataract proof.

If you have cataracts, there are various alternative treatments to get rid of them, including electromagnetic treatment, homeopathic remedies, herbal treatments, and N-acetyl-carnosine drops in the eyes twice daily. Cataracts are easily prevented and can be reversed—no need for surgery.

Anti-Aging Medicine Accelerates Aging

Aging, as we experience it in the West, is nothing but a disease of accumulated repair deficits. Whether our aging shows up as wrinkled skin, joint problems, or a chronic disease, the truth is that we age systemically, and fixing one outward sign of aging or another will never prevent or reverse aging. The root causes of our premature aging are deficiency and toxicity—and the way to stay biologically young is to correct both of these through the Six Pathways I have described in this book.

Conventional medicine treats aging as it does all disease—with instant mechanistic solutions, substituting surgery, drugs, and devices for the body's own repair systems. Not only does this approach not facilitate repairs, it destroys the very mechanisms that make it possible for our cells to repair and rejuvenate themselves. Older Americans are spending billions of dollars on prescription drugs, hormone replacement therapies, and elective surgery. What they are buying is cellular malfunction, accelerated aging, and more disease.

HRT Crashes Your Endocrine System

Hormone replacement therapy (HRT) is another way conventional medicine does irreparable harm. Numerous studies have proven that HRT causes heart attack, stroke, and blood clots. It does this because it disturbs the delicate balance of hormones in the body, and that accelerates the aging process. Women on HRT are up to three times more likely to develop blood clots as well as cancer. After decades of well-founded suspicion, it has now been established that HRT causes cancer. A study of 46,000 women in a 2000 issue of the *Journal of the American Medical Association* found that women who used the most common form of HRT for five years had a 40 percent increased risk of breast cancer, and that the risk increased by 8 percent with each year of use. A 2010 study in the *Journal of the American Medical Association* found that not only does HRT increase the risk of breast cancer, but it also makes it more likely the cancer will be aggressive and deadly. In addition to breast cancer, a 2006 study in the *Journal of the National Cancer Institute* found a link between HRT and ovarian cancer; other studies have found links to lung cancer. Since 2000, many physicians have stopped prescribing HRT, and studies show that the recent decline in breast cancer deaths is the direct result of that change. Fewer patients are dying from breast cancer because fewer doctors are giving them cancer!

While traditional hormone replacement therapy was a disaster, it used molecules that were not natural to the human body. These hormones were synthetic or derived from animals. Today, a number of alternative physicians are using hormone therapy with molecules that are, supposedly, biologically identical to molecules used by the body. However, bioidentical hormones are not really identical to human hormones. They are similar, but not identical, and there is no long-term proof of their safety. Nevertheless, current evidence indicates that bioidentical hormones, when properly used, are associated with lower risks than traditional HRT. Lower risk does not mean no risk. Any form of drug therapy has associated risks, and these risks have to be balanced against the benefits.

Prescription Lenses Can Ruin Eyesight

It's a commonly held belief that eyesight inevitably gets worse with age and that glasses are the only solution when it happens. However, prescription lenses, especially when stronger than needed, may be doing more than just helping you keep your driver's license. They may accelerate your vision loss.

Presbyopia, also known as "aging eyes," causes near objects to look blurry and occurs because our eyes have lost their strength and agility, and hence their ability to shift focus. This is a direct result of the way we habitually use our eyes over time. Early in human evolution, when we lived most of our lives in the great outdoors, eyes were constantly adjusting to various perspectives—focusing far into the distance as well as on objects close at hand. All the eye muscles got their fair share of exercise. But these days we over-focus on close-range tasks, like reading and computer work, and our eyes become fixed in one position.

Prescription glasses correct this lack of focus, but in a way that actually increases the rigid way in which we use our eyes. Lenses that are stronger than needed are especially bad. To maintain vision, we need the exact opposite—more varied eye use that exercises all of our eye muscles in a balanced way.

The good news is that many people have regained the clear eyesight of their youth with vision training—specific exercises that relax and exercise eye muscles in a therapeutic way. Although there is a time commitment involved, vision training does not involve any expensive equipment or invasive procedures, and the results can be quite remarkable, even correcting astigmatism.

Conventional Dentistry Fills You with Toxins

Conventional dentistry uses X-rays, toxic metals such as nickel and mercury, and carcinogenic local anesthetics. It is widely acknowledged that there is no safe level of radiation, yet dentists use X-rays routinely. Another routine dental procedure, the root canal, allows dangerous disease-causing bacteria to breed in your mouth. Let's have a look at some of the problems:

Fillings

A so-called silver filling actually consists of about 50 percent liquid mercury mixed with powdered silver, tin, and copper. Despite the fact that mercury is one of the most dangerous toxins in our environment, damaging the brain, central nervous system, immune system, and kidneys, as well as causing cancer, an estimated 100 million mercury fillings are still done each year in the United States. There is no safe level of mercury. The EPA recommends that we ingest no more than a maximum of 0.1 micrograms per kilogram of body weight per day. This translates to no more than 6.8 micrograms of mercury per day for a 150-pound person. Average daily absorption from fish and seafood is estimated at 2.3 micrograms. Alarmingly, a single mercury filling, through evaporation and mechanical wear, can release 15 micrograms per day, every day. A person with eight fillings will be absorbing 120 micrograms per day. Fortunately, plastic composites are now used extensively in place of the mercury fillings. Anyone with mercury fillings should have them removed, but it must be done by a dentist who has the necessary equipment and follows the specific procedures required for safe removal—you should have your own air supply during the removal so as not to breathe the mercury vapors. For more information and to find a dentist qualified to do safe removal of mercury fillings, go to the website of the International Academy of Oral Medicine and Toxicology, *www.iaomt.org.*

Crowns

About 75 percent of porcelain crowns are made with a stainless steel liner to give them strength. The stainless contains nickel. Nickel is an allergen and is an even more powerful carcinogen than mercury. If you have porcelain crowns made with nickel, it would be best to remove them. Crowns made with gold are a better choice. Today porcelain technology has advanced to where crowns are available that have no metal at all; these would be the best choice.

Root Canals

Even though for more than a century scientists have been warning of the dangers of endodontic therapy (commonly referred to as a "root canal"), conventional dentistry still considers it safe. Yet in virtually every tooth on which this procedure is performed, dead tissue is left behind that is highly susceptible to infection. These low-grade infections produce toxins that poison the entire body, damaging immunity. Endodontically treated teeth are breeding grounds for highly toxic bacteria. A strong immune system will keep the infection in check. But once your immunity has been compromised, the bacteria can migrate into the bloodstream and infect any organ, gland, or tissue. Removal of the diseased tooth is the only safe option.

Unfortunately, few dentists recognize the serious long-lasting risks of root canals. There is no data to prove that endodontic therapy is safe. Meanwhile, there is mounting evidence to the contrary, starting with the pioneering research of Dr. Weston A. Price.

In the early 1900s, Dr. Price discovered that root-canalled teeth become infected with bacteria and that they are responsible for many chronic diseases, the most frequent being heart disease. To prove his point, Dr. Price famously implanted fragments of endodontically treated human teeth into rabbits. The healthy animals soon developed the same conditions as the human donor.

Heart disease, kidney disease, arthritis, neurological and autoimmune diseases—nearly every chronic degenerative disease can result from a root canal, years or decades after the procedure.

Dr. Price published his research in 1922. Unfortunately, his work went mostly unrecognized for seventy years, until root canal specialist Dr. George Meinig rediscovered it. In 1993, Meinig published his own book, *Root Canal Cover-Up,* a comprehensive reference on this topic.

Some dentists will recommend an implant. As a general rule don't put things in your body that don't belong there. The titanium alloy used for dental implants can cause allergic or inflammatory reactions in some people. Bacteria and viruses tend to target implants, putting stress on your immune system. In addition, about one-third of all nerve injuries caused by dental work have been associated with implants, resulting in constant pain or numbness. It is best to remove the tooth and put in a partial.

Anesthetics

Local anesthetics, such as lidocaine, are commonly used by dentists. These chemicals break down in the body into cancer-causing compounds called anilines. In 1993, the FDA found that lidocaine, when exposed to human tissue, breaks down into 2,6-dimethylaniline, a compound that is known to cause cancer. In September 1996, because of these findings, the FDA removed from the market all over-the-counter painkillers containing these local anesthetics and required that a warning be placed on all new prescription pharmaceuticals containing them. Unfortunately, preexisting prescription anesthetics were not required to carry the FDA's warning, and most health professionals are still unaware of this problem. Fortunately, there is a new anesthetic that is not cancer causing—Septocaine. You can request that your dentist use this product.

In Conclusion

The health care system in America needs serious rethinking. Our century old, conventional allopathic medicine is fatally flawed and has become a major cause of disease and our leading cause of death. It has failed to keep abreast of the enormous advances in science over the last century, or to put these discoveries into clinical practice. The health care delivery system has become corrupted by multinational drug, insurance, and food industry interests that put their profits ahead of your health. It is a system that relies on treating only the symptoms of disease and never the causes. The reason health care costs so much is that conventional medicine doesn't cure anybody. Patients stay sick while money is spent to manage their symptoms and to cope with the harm done by their treatments.

The way to cure any disease is to restore malfunctioning cells to normal by addressing the two causes of disease: deficiency and toxicity. When making health care choices for yourself or your loved ones, keep these facts in mind. The best approach is to keep yourself in good health. Keep your immunity strong by eating a good diet, taking high-quality supplements, and avoiding environmental toxins, prescription drugs, vaccinations, and antibiotics.

The Bottom Line

✓ Although conventional medicine excels at crisis intervention and trauma care, it is not only unhelpful but dangerous when it comes to dealing with aging and chronic degenerative disease. Use the information in this book to address the true causes of accelerated aging and disease, and protect yourself from an outdated medical system that can be hazardous to your health.

✓ Screening is not prevention, and many diagnostic tests actually cause disease or make disease worse. No level of ionizing radiation is safe, and mammograms and CT scans expose you to ionizing radiation. Even needle biopsies have been known to spread cancer. Thermography is vastly superior to mammography for detecting breast cancer. While mammograms have high percentages of false negatives and false positives, thermography can detect breast cancer by up to a decade earlier with no false negatives and few false positives, and without radiation.

✓ All pharmaceutical drugs are toxic. They interfere with normal cell function—the definition of toxicity. Most drugs cause nutrient deficiencies as well. Avoid taking drugs. If you already take them, find a competent health care practitioner who can help you gradually wean yourself off of them. If you are considering taking any of the following—cholesterol drugs, birth control pills, TNF blockers, antibiotics, and flu shots or other vaccinations—please review the relevant sections in this chapter.

✓ Surgeries are damaging and aging at best, dangerous at worst. They should never be performed unless absolutely necessary and there is no other alternative. However, there is almost always an alternative (an estimated ninety percent of all surgeries are unnecessary). See sections in this chapter on heart bypass, hip implant, and cataract surgeries and what to do instead.

✓ Conventional hormone replacement has been shown to cause heart attacks, blood clots, strokes, and cancer. Bioidentical hormones are similar to human hormones, but not identical, and there is no long-term proof that they are safe. Current evidence indicates they pose less risk than conventional hormone replacement; but less risk is not the same as no risk.

✓ It is commonly believed that vision gets worse with age, making eyeglasses inevitable. Actually it is the way we use our eyes— overusing them for short-range vision—that worsens vision. Although it takes a commitment of time, eye exercises can prevent and correct vision problems. Prescription eyeglasses, on the other hand, especially when stronger than needed, can make your eyesight worse.

✓ Conventional dentistry is a potential source of dangerous toxicity. Decline all dental X-rays unless absolutely necessary. Avoid "silver" dental fillings (which are actually 50 percent mercury) and have such fillings removed by a dentist who has received special training to do this type of work. If you need crowns, choose all-porcelain crowns without metal. About 75 percent of porcelain crowns contain nickel—an allergen and potent carcinogen. Avoid root canals. If you need a dental anesthetic, choose Septocaine. Other dental anesthetics break down in the body into cancer-causing compounds.

CHAPTER 10

Now What?

Knowing is not enough; we must apply.
Willing is not enough; we must do.

—Johann Wolfgang von Goethe

It is not only what we do,
but also what we do not do, for which
we are accountable.

—Molière

I T HAS BEEN SAID THAT KNOWLEDGE IS POWER. If so, you have just become a very powerful person. Congratulations! You now know more than the average medical doctor about how to achieve health, prevent disease, and slow the aging process.

You have just learned a revolutionary, yet simple, approach to health and disease that is so powerful, it can be used to prevent and reverse almost all disease. You now know that while there are thousands of symptoms, there is *only one disease*. You know what disease is: *malfunctioning cells*. You know what causes cells to malfunction: *deficiency and toxicity*. You also know how to prevent and cure disease: *by eliminating deficiency and toxicity and restoring cells to normal function*. You also know why our society is experiencing an epidemic of accelerated aging, why it is a mistake, and how to prevent and even reverse this unnecessary and destructive type of aging.

Armed with this cutting-edge knowledge, the question becomes this: What are you going to do with it? Knowledge has no value until you put it into action. There is a big difference between knowing something and doing something about it. For example, 95 percent of Americans believe that wearing a seatbelt would help protect them in an accident, yet only 69 percent of Americans wear seatbelts. We don't always do what we know is best.

Then again, we don't always know what is best. Often this is due to an abundance of misinformation and the marginalization of good information by powerful moneyed interests that are much more focused on quarterly earnings than on your health and well-being. We are subjected daily to a blizzard of advertising messages about what we should eat and what medicines we should ask our doctor about. These ads are not based on scientific data about what supports your body in maintaining health. They are designed solely to increase the profits of the advertisers. As a result, most of us are eating "foods" and taking medications that rob us of our health, so disease is rampant in our society.

To make matters worse, we then look to our doctors to fix the problems that we have created. But they are of little help because most physicians have been taught an obsolete, unscientific concept of disease. They do not understand what disease is, why it happens, or how to cure it—*but you do!* You have been provided with a roadmap to a long, productive, disease-free life. This roadmap consists of the Six Pathways to better health and graceful aging. All you have to do is use them. Yet we are all prone to procrastination. Institutions, governments, and businesses often do things that are not in your best interest, so you have to take responsibility for your own health and not delegate it to these entities. I have given you the tools you need, but the next step is up to you.

What's Stopping You?

Nothing has ever been more resisted in human experience than a new idea. Yet you need to put the new ideas you have just learned into action. You cannot continue to eat the same diet, expose yourself to the same toxins, and live the same lifestyle and expect better results. Change is necessary. Without our society making massive changes, we are doomed to experience an increasingly sick population, more accelerated aging, and costs that are certain to bankrupt our nation.

Some of you will resist change because you feel overwhelmed. Once you understand how massively our food supply and environment have been compromised, you may feel discouraged and just give up. But every great journey starts with the first step. Even if you don't do it all, there are simple changes anyone can make that have a big payoff. For example, sugar is a deadly metabolic poison that will age you and make you sick. *Get sugar out of your life. Eat more fresh, organic produce. Use safe household and personal care products. Don't take prescription drugs.* These are simple changes, and they have a big payoff. Why not do them?

Consider that most of us are unhealthy because we are doing most things wrong most of the time, thereby accelerating the aging process. Turn that around and do most things right most of the time; it will be like a miracle. You don't have to be perfect!

Many people don't change because they are fearful of what others will think if they are different. You want to fit in with the others and go with the flow. Yet there is much to be said for leadership and showing others the way by example. It's not easy to break with tradition and to be the first to be different, but people around the world have thanked me for improving and even saving their lives through my example. I remember decades ago when people thought I was odd because of what I chose to eat or not eat. But many of the choices I made back then are now becoming widely accepted. Many people have told me that I was far ahead of the crowd. I got the Big Four out of my life. I simply don't eat sugar, wheat, processed oils, or milk products. I had to make drastic changes to save my life, and then to take myself from near death to superior health. The results speak for themselves. Now people are eager to know what I eat and what supplements I take, so they can do the same and enjoy the level of health and vitality that I enjoy. Our society needs change, and for that, we need leaders to show the way—you can be one.

Many people I encounter don't change because they don't see the need. They think they are healthy. I have had cancer patients tell me that, other than their cancer, they are in perfect health. This is delusional. If you have a disease, it is because you are sick, not because you are healthy. Many people with diabetes and obese people have told me they are in good health. They obviously don't know what health is. Any disease affects the entire body. Less than 1 percent of the U.S. population is healthy; the remainder is in some stage of disease. We can and must turn this around. We really don't have a choice, because our epidemic of chronic disease is bankrupting us. You can help by first turning yourself around. Your superior health, vitality, and youthful appearance will become an inspiration to those around you.

Another reason people don't change—even when they want to—is a lack of urgency. If you have been injured, you may not know what to do, but you will surely do something, because the situation is urgent. When you keep eating the wrong foods and gaining weight, you are just as surely injuring yourself, but the difference is there is no sense of urgency. We all have a "normalcy bias," a tendency to expect things today to be the same as yesterday, even if there is gradually mounting evidence that things are changing. So you may need to create your own sense of urgency. Give yourself some deadlines to motivate you to act. It really is more urgent than it seems for you to take action to improve your health and avoid aging prematurely.

Make Health a Habit

We are all creatures of habit, and food rituals such as that late-night bowl of ice cream or those mid-afternoon cookies may give us momentary comfort, even though they challenge our health. But we can break these habits and acquire new ones—healthy habits. For most of us, it's best to do this gradually, making incremental improvements over time. This makes the changes seem more achievable and reduces the stress of trying to do it all at once. For example, you might take on the Big Four one at a time. One friend declared to himself and others, "I'm having a wheat-free May," and then committed to avoid anything with wheat in it for the next thirty days. He found that easier than saying, "I will never eat wheat again." At the end of that month, he was so pleased with his visibly smaller belly that he continued to avoid wheat. More than a year later, his physique and his digestive health are much improved.

Another approach is to eliminate foods that contain two or more of the Big Four. For example, to eliminate both sugar and wheat from your diet, start with products that contain both sugar and wheat, such as cookies and cakes. To eliminate both sugar and dairy, start by eliminating ice cream.

It is important to reward yourself for your small successes. Give yourself a pat on the back whenever you stick with your good intentions and overcome a temptation. But don't beat yourself up when you do backslide—it's bound to happen from time to time. The guilt you feel could actually be more damaging to your health than the occasional slip-up, so don't be hard on yourself! Stay positive and focus on what you're doing right, not what you're doing wrong.

Set some goals for yourself, and as you are increasingly success-ful in making positive changes, give yourself a reward. Buy that nice thing you have been wanting, go out for a night on the town, or take that special vacation. This will help to reinforce your new habits and strengthen your willingness to continue making changes.

Get Well, Stay Well, and . . . Never Feel Old Again

Aging results from lack of maintenance and the body's accumu-lation of repair deficits—the same way your car ages. Accelerated aging is a disease process that accelerates the accumulation of repair deficits. To stop this process, you must get well and stay well. Start getting well by eliminating foods with little nutritional value and replacing them with nutrient-dense foods. Think before you eat. *With each mouthful of food, you are choosing either to support cel-lular repair and delay the aging process, or to create repair deficits and accelerate aging.* Get packaged, processed foods out of your diet. As you are getting these toxic foods out, start putting more fresh whole fruits and vegetables in, preferably organic. Remember, you are eating to give your cells what they need to repair themselves and function normally. If they don't get what they need, you *will* get sick—guaranteed!

Get the toxins out of your life. Filter your air and water. Stop using toxic personal care products, such as toxic toothpaste. Avoid toxic prescription and over-the-counter drugs and vaccinations. Nutritionally support your detoxification systems, and detoxify using frequent saunas. Think positively and follow a spiritual practice. Be sure to get regular exercise, sunlight, and adequate sleep. Avoid chronic noise and electromagnetic fields. Protect your DNA from toxic or radiation damage and support your DNA repair systems with good nutrition. Avoid medical procedures that are not absolutely necessary to address some crisis.

Get yourself moving in the right direction on the Six Pathways, choose to put purpose and joy in your life, and you will almost certainly live longer, healthier, and happier, without the disability caused by accelerated aging.

Wishing you good health and long life,
Raymond Francis

REFERENCES

Age-Related Eye Disease Study Research Group. "A randomized, placebo-controlled, clinical trial of high-dose supplementation with vitamins C and E, beta carotene, and zinc for age-related macular degeneration and vision loss: AREDS report no. 8." *Archives of Ophthalmology* (2001) 119 (10): 1417–36.

Alford, L. "What men should know about the impact of physical activity on their health." *International Journal of Clinical Practice* (2010) 64 (13): 1731.

Allen, M. "Assembly-line colonoscopies at clinic described." *Las Vegas Sun*, http://www.lasvegassun.com/news/2008/mar/09/assembly-line-colonoscopies-clinic-described/.

American Cancer Society. "American Cancer Society Guidelines for the Early Detection of Cancer," http://www.cancer.org/healthy/findcancerearly/cancerscreeningguidelines/american-cancer-society-guidelines-for-the-early-detection-of-cancer.

Ames, B. "Micronutrients Prevent Cancer and Delay Aging," a paper presented at the meeting at the Strang International Cancer Prevention Conference in New York City, 1998.

———. "Micronutrient deficiencies: A major cause of DNA damage." *Annals of the New York Academy of Sciences* (1999) 889 (1): 87–106.

Anderson, R. "Toxic emissions from carpets." *Journal of Nutritional and Environmental Medicine* 5 (1995): 375–86.

Andrew, B., et al. "Meditation effects on cognitive function and cerebral blood flow in subjects with memory loss: A preliminary study." *Journal of Alzheimer's Disease* (2010) 20 (2): 517–26.

Angell, M. *The Truth About the Drug Companies: How They Deceive Us and What to Do About It.* New York: Random House, 2005.

Aris, A., and Leblanc, S. "Maternal and fetal exposure to pesticides associated to genetically modified foods in Eastern Townships of Quebec, Canada." *Reproductive Toxicology* (2011) 31 (4): 528–33.

Armanios, M., et. al. "Short telomeres are sufficient to cause the degenerative defects associated with aging." *American Journal of Human Genetics* (2009) 85 (6): 823–32.

Armstrong, B., and Doll, R. "Environmental factors and cancer incidence and mortality in different countries with special reference to dietary practices." *International Journal of Cancer* (1975) 15 (4): 617–31.

Arnetz, B.B., et al. "The effects of 884 MHz GSM wireless communication signals on self-reported symptom and sleep (EEG): An experimental provocation study." *PIERS Online* (2007) 3 (7): 1148–50.

Auso, E., et al. "A moderate and transient deficiency of maternal thyroid function at the beginning of fetal neocorticogenesis alters neuronal migration." *Endocrinology* (2004) 145 (9): 4037–47.

Baillie-Hamilton, P. *Toxic Overload.* New York: Avery, Penguin, 2005.

Barbagallo, M., et al. "Magnesium homeostasis and aging." *Magnesium Research* (2009) 22 (4): 235–46.

Barclay, R.L., et al. "Colonoscopic withdrawal times and adenoma detection during screening colonoscopy." *New England Journal of Medicine* (2006) 355 (24): 2533–41.

Bebeshko, V., et al. "Does ionizing radiation accelerate the aging phenomena?" *International Conference: Twenty Years after Chernobyl Accident, Future Outlook.* April 24–26, 2006, Kiev, Ukraine. Contributed Papers (HOLTEH, Kiev), 1:13–18.

Becker, R.O., and Selden, G. *The Body Electric: Electromagnetism and the Foundation of Life.* New York: William Morrow, 1985.

Beecher, H. K. "The powerful placebo." *Journal of the American Medical Association* (1959) 159: 1602–6.

Blair, S. N., et al. "The Fitness, Obesity, and Health Equation." *Journal of the American Medical Association,* September 8, 2004: 1232–34.

Berkrot, B., and Pierson, R. "FDA adds diabetes, memory loss warnings to statins." Reuters, http://www.reuters.com/article/2012/02/28/us-fda-statins-idUSTRE81R1O220120228.

Bernstein, I.L., et al. "Immune responses in farm workers after exposure to Bacillus thuringiensis pesticides." *Environmental Health Perspectives* (1999) 107 (7): 575–82.

Bibbins-Domingo, K., et al. "Projected effect of dietary salt reductions on future cardiovascular disease." *New England Journal of Medicine* (2010) 362 (7): 590–99.

Bieler, H. *Food Is Your Best Medicine.* New York: Ballantine Books, 1987.

Bjornberg, K.A., et al. "Methylmercury exposure in Swedish women with high fish consumption." *Science of the Total Environment* (2003) 342 (1–3): 45–52.

Blaylock, R. L., MD. *Excitotoxins.* Santa Fe, NM: Health Press, 1997.

———. *Health and Nutrition Secrets that Can Save Your Life.* Albuquerque, NM: Health Press, 2002.

———. *Natural Strategies for Cancer Patients.* New York, NY: Kensington, 2003.

Bloom, M., et al. "Environmental exposure to PBDEs and thyroid function among New York anglers." *Environmental Toxicology and Pharmacology* (2007) 25 (3): 386–92.

Bocio, A., et al. "Polybrominated diphenyl ethers (DBDEs) in foodstuffs: Human exposure through diet." *Journal of Agricultural Food Chemistry* (2003) 51 (10): 3191–95.

Bone, E., et al. "The production of urinary phenols by gut bacteria and their possible role in the causation of large bowel cancer." *American Journal of Clinical Nutrition* (1976) 29 (12): 1448–54.

Bonita, R., et al. "Changes in stroke incidence and case-fatality in Auckland, New Zealand, 1981–91." *Lancet* (1993) 342 (8885): 1470–73.

Boutwell, R.K., and Bosch, D.K. "The tumor-promoting action of phenol and related compounds for mouse skin." *Cancer Research* (1959) 19: 413–24.

Bowman, G.L., et al. "Nutrient biomarker patterns, cognitive function, and MRI measures of brain aging." *Neurology* (2012) 78 (4): 241–49.

Brassen, S., et al. "Anterior cingulate activation is related to a positivity bias and emotional stability in successful aging." *Biological Psychiatry* (2011) 70 (2): 131–37.

Brenner, D.J., and Elliston, C.D. "Estimated radiation risks potentially associated with full-body CT screening." *Radiology* (2004) 232 (3): 735–38.

Brinton, L.A., et al. "Oral contraceptives and breast cancer risk among younger women." *Journal of the National Cancer Institute* (1995) 87 (13): 827–35.

Brouilette, S.W., et al. "Telomere length, risk of coronary heart disease, and statin treatment in the West of Scotland Primary Prevention Study: A nested case-control study." *Lancet* (2007) 369 (9556): 81–82.

Burton, G.W., et al. "Human plasma and tissue alpha-tocopherol concentrations in response to supplementation with deuterated natural and synthetic vitamin E." *American Journal of Clinical Nutrition* (1998) 67 (4): 669–84.

Buxton, J.L., et al. "Childhood obesity is associated with shorter leukocyte telomere length." *Journal of Clinical Endocrinology and Metabolism* (2011) 96 (5): 1500–1505.

Canela, A., et al. "High-throughput telomere length quantification by FISH and its application to human population studies." *Proceedings of the National Academy of Sciences* (2007) 104 (13): 5300–5305.

Carlton, R. Quoted from *Marketplace*, Canadian Broadcast Company, November 24, 1992.

Casey, B.M., et al. "Subclinical hyperthyroidism and pregnancy outcomes." *Obstetrics and Gynecology* (2006) 107 (2 Pt 1): 337–41.

Cawthon, R.M., et al. "Association between telomere length in blood and mortality in people aged 60 years or older." *Lancet* (2003) 361 (9355): 393–95.

Centers for Disease Control. *Childhood Obesity Facts.* Accessed on March 12, 2013, http://www.cdc.gov/healthyyouth/obesity/facts.htm.

Centers for Disease Control. *Fourth National Report on Human Exposure to Environmental Chemicals.* National Institutes of Health, 2009.

Chan, J.M., et al. "Dairy products, calcium, and prostate cancer risk in the Physicians' Health Study." *American Journal of Clinical Nutrition* (2001) 74 (4): 549–54.

Chen, C.L., et al. "Hormone replacement therapy in relation to breast cancer." *Journal of the American Medical Association* (2002) 287 (6): 734–41.

Cherkas, L., et al. "The association between physical activity in leisure time and leukocyte telomere length." *Archives of Internal Medicine* (2008) 168 (2): 154–58.

Chevrier, J., et al. "Associations between prenatal exposure to polychlorinated biphenyls and neonatal thyroid-stimulating hormone levels in a Mexican-American population, Salinas Valley, California." *Environmental Health Perspectives* (2007) 115 (10): 1490–96.

Chien, L.C., et al. "Hair mercury concentration and fish consumption: Risk and perception of risk among women of childbearing age." *Environmental Research* (2010) 110 (1): 123–29.

Chlebowski, R.T., et al. "Estrogen plus progestin and breast cancer incidence and mortality in postmenopausal women." *Journal of the American Medical Association* (2010) 304 (15): 1684–92.

Chopra, D. *Quantum Healing.* New York: Bantam New Age Books, 1990.

Christensen, K., et al. "Perceived age as clinically useful biomarker of ageing: Cohort study." *British Medical Journal* (2009) 339: b5262.

Clarke, J.D. *Prostate cancer prevention with broccoli: From cellular to human studies.* Ann Arbor, MI: ProQuest, UMI Dissertation Publishing, 2012.

Clinton, S.K., et al. "Effects of ammonium acetate and sodium cholate on N-methyl-N'-nitro-N-nitrosoguanidine-induced colon carcinogenesis of rats." *Cancer Research* (1988) 48 (11): 3035–39.

Colagar, A.H. "Zinc levels in seminal plasma are associated with sperm quality in fertile and infertile men." *Nutritional Research* (2009) 29 (2): 82–88.

Colbert, D. *Toxic Relief: Restore Health and Energy Through Fasting and Detoxification.* Lake Mary, FL: Siloam, 2003.

Cologne, J.B., and Preston, D.L. "Longevity of atomic-bomb survivors." *Lancet* (2000) 356 (9226): 303–7.

Committee on Quality of Health Care in America and Institute of Medicine. *Crossing the Quality Chasm: A New Health System for the 21st Century.* Washington, DC: National Academies Press, 2001.

Comstock, G.W., and Partridge, K.B. "Church attendance and health." *Journal of Chronic Disease* (1972) 25 (12): 665–72.

Congcong, H., et al. "Exercise-induced BCL2-regulated autophagy is required for muscle glucose homeostasis." *Nature* (2012) 481 (7382): 511–15.

Consumer Reports. "Wrinkle creams: Miracle or mirage?" http://www.consumerreports.org/cro/magazine-archive/2011/september/health/wrinkle-creams/overview/index.htm.

Corpet, D.E., et al. "Colonic protein fermentation and promotion of colon carcinogenesis by thermolyzed casein." *Nutrition and Cancer* (1995) 23 (3): 271–81.

———. "Promotion of colonic microadenoma growth in mice and rats fed cooked sugar or cooked casein and fat." *Cancer Research* (1990) 50 (21): 6955–58.

Costello L.C., et al. "Decreased zinc and downregulation of ZIP3 zinc uptake transporter in the development of pancreatic adenocarcinoma." *Cancer Biology and Therapy* (2011) 12 (4): 297–303.

Costenbader, K.H., et al. "Immunosenescence and rheumatoid arthritis: Does telomere shortening predict impending disease?" *Autoimmunity Reviews* (2011) 10 (9): 569–73.

Crary, D. "Boomers will be spending billions to counter aging." *USA Today,* http://usatoday30.usatoday.com/news/health/story/health/story/2011/08/Anti-aging-industry-grows-with-boomer-demand/50087672/1.

Dallaire, R., et al. "Thyroid function and plasma concentrations of polyhalogenated compounds in Inuit adults." *Environmental Health Perspectives* (2009) 117 (9): 1380–86.

Davis, P.A., et al. "Walnuts reduce prostate tumor size and growth in a mouse model of prostate cancer." American Chemical Society spring national meeting, San Francisco, California. Abstract #59, Agricultural and Food Chemistry Division, March 22, 2010.

Dean, C. *Death by Modern Medicine*. New York: Matrix Verite Media, 2005.

Deardorff, J. "What berries can do for you." *Chicago Tribune News*, http://articles.chicagotribune.com/2011-03-02/health/sc-health-0302-berries-health-effects20110302_1_blueberries-bladder-infections-health-benefits.

Dei Cas, A., et al. "Lower endothelial progenitor cell number, family history of cardiovascular disease and reduced HDL-cholesterol levels are associated with shorter leukocyte telomere length in healthy young adults." *Nutrition, Metabolism, and Cardiovascular Diseases* (2011).

Devore, E.E., et al. "Dietary intakes of berries and flavonoids in relation to cognitive decline." *Annals of Neurology* (2012) 72 (1): 135–43.

———. "Relative telomere length and cognitive decline in the Nurses' Health Study." *Neuroscience Letters* (2011) 492 (1): 15–18.

Diamond, H. *Fit for Life: A New Beginning*. New York: Kensington Books, 2000.

Diez, S., et al. "Prenatal and early childhood exposure to mercury and methylmercury in Spain, a high fish consumer country." *Archives of Environmental Contamination and Toxicology* (2009) 56 (3): 615–22.

Disabled World. "Average life span expectancy chart—How long will I live," http://www.disabled-world.com/calculators-charts/life-expectancy-statistics.php.

Dolecek, T.A., and Grandits, G. "Dietary polyunsaturated fatty acids and mortality in the Multiple Risk Factor Intervention Trial (MRFIT). "*World Review of Nutrition and Dietetics* (1991) 66: 205–16.

Dossey, L. *The Power of Prayer and the Practice of Medicine.* San Francisco, CA: Harper, 1993.

Du, M., et al. "Physical activity, sedentary behavior, and leukocyte telomere length in women." *American Journal of Epidemiology* (2012) 175 (5): 414–22.

Dufault, R., et al. "Mercury from chlor-alkali plants: Measured concentrations in food product sugar." *Environmental Health* (2009) 8 (1): 2.

Edwards, J. "Lawsuit claims Pfizer deceived doctors into prescribing its cholesterol drug Lipitor." *CBS News*, http://www.cbsnews.com/8301-505123_162-42844207/lawsuit-claims-pfizer-deceived-doctors-into-prescribing-its-cholesterol-drug-lipitor/.

Eger, H., et al. "The influence of being physically near to a cell phone transmission mast on the incidence of cancer." *Umwelt Medizin Gesellschaft* (2004) 17 (4): 326–32.

Ehrlich, S.D. "Acne." University of Marland Medical Center, http://www.umm.edu/altmed/articles/acne-000001.htm.

Environmental Working Group. "Chromium-6 is widespread in US tap water," http://www.ewg.org/chromium6-in-tap-water.

———. "Testing finds hundreds of contaminants in America's drinking water," http://www.ewg.org/tap-water/reportfindings.

Epel, E.S., et al. "Accelerated telomere shortening in response to life stress." *Proceedings of the National Academy of Sciences* (2004) 101 (49): 17312–15.

Epstein, L.J., and Mardon, S. *The Harvard Medical School Guide to a Good Night's Sleep.* New York: McGraw Hill, 2006.

Erasmus, U. *Fats and Oils.* Vancouver, Canada: Alive Books, 1986.

Escrich, E., et al. "Olive oil, an essential component of the Mediterranean diet, and breast cancer." *Public Health Nutrition* (2011) 14 (12): 2323–32.

Espel, E., et al. "The rate of leukocyte telomere shortening predicts mortality from cardiovascular disease in elderly men." *AGING* (2008) 1 (1): 81–88.

Fallon, S., with Enig, M.G. *Nourishing Traditions: The Cookbook that Challenges Politically Correct Nutrition and the Diet Dictocrats.* Washington, DC: New Trends, 2000.

Fälth-Magnusson, K., and Mangusson, K.E. "Elevated levels of serum antibodies to the lectin wheat germ agglutinin in celiac children lend support to the gluten-lectin theory of celiac disease." *Pediatric Allergy and Immunology* (1995) 6 (2): 98–102.

Farzaneh-Far, R., et al. "Association of marine omega-3 fatty acid levels with telomeric gaining in patients with coronary heart disease." *Journal of the American Medical Association* (2010) 303 (3): 250–57.

Finamore, A., et al. "Intestinal and peripheral immune response to MON810 maize ingestion in weaning and old mice." *Journal of Agricultural and Food Chemistry* (2008) 56 (23): 11533–39.

Fowler, S., et al. "Diet soft drink consumption is associated with increased waist circumference in the San Antonio Longitudinal Study of Aging," an abstract presented at the annual meeting of the American Diabetes Association in San Diego, California, Abstract No. 62-OR, 2011.

Francis, R. *Never Be Fat Again.* Deerfield Beach, FL: Health Communications, Inc., 2007.

———. *Never Be Sick Again.* Deerfield Beach, FL: Health Communications, Inc., 2002.

———. *Never Fear Cancer Again*. Deerfield Beach, FL: Health Communications, Inc., 2011.

Friedman, H.S., et al. "Personality and health, subjective well-being, and longevity." *Journal of Personality* (2010) 78: 179–215.

Friedman, M., et al. "Reactions of proteins with dehydroalanines." *Advances in Experimental Medicine and Biology* (1975) 86B: 213–24.

Gardener, H., et al. "Diet soft drink consumption is associated with an increased risk of vascular events in the Northern Manhattan Study." *Journal of General Internal Medicine* (2012) 27 (9): 1120–26.

George, M.G., et al. "Trends in stroke hospitalizations and associated risk factors among children and young adults, 1995–2008." *Annals of Neurology* (2011) 70 (5): 713–21.

Green, J. Citizens for Safe Drinking Water. Accessed on March 11, 2013. http://www.keepers-of-the-well.org

Godfrey, R.J., et al. "The exercise-induced growth hormone response in athletes." *Sports Medicine* (2003) 33 (8): 599–613.

Gofman, J.W. *Radiation from Medical Procedures in the Pathogenesis of Cancer and Ischemic Heart Disease: Dose-Response Studies with Physicians per 100,000 Population*. San Francisco: Committee for Nuclear Responsibility, 1999.

Golomb, B. "Effects of statins on energy and fatigue with exertion: Results from a randomized controlled trial." *Archives of Internal Medicine* (2012) 172 (15): 1180–82.

———. "Statin adverse effects: A review of the literature and evidence for a mitochondrial mechanism." *American Journal of Cardiovascular Drugs* (2008) 8 (6): 373–418.

Griffiths, D., and Sturm, J. "Epidemiology and etiology of young stroke." *Stroke Research and Treatment* 2011 (2011): Article ID 209370.

Guzyeyeva, G.V. "Lectin glycosylation as a marker of thin gut inflammation." *FASEB Journal* (2008) 22: 898.3.

Haddow, J.E., et al. "Maternal thyroid deficiency during pregnancy and subsequent neuropsychological development of the child." *New England Journal of Medicine* (1999) 341 (8): 549–55.

Hadler, N.M. "Knee pain is the malady—not osteoarthritis." *Annals of Internal Medicine* (1992) 116 (7): 598–99.

Halldorsson, T.I., et al. "Intake of artificially sweetened soft drinks and risk of preterm delivery: A prospective cohort study in 59,334 Danish pregnant women." *American Journal of Clinical Nutrition* (2010) 92 (3): 626–33.

Harbige, L. "Fatty acids, the immune response, and autoimmunity: A question of n-6 essentiality and the balance between n-6 and n-3." *Lipids* (2003) 38 (4): 323–41.

Harley, C.B., et al. "A natural product telomerase activator as part of a health maintenance program." *Rejuvenation Research* (2011) 14 (1): 45–56.

Harley, K.G., et al. "PBDE concentrations in women's serum and fecundability." *Environmental Health Perspectives* (2010) 118 (5): 699–704.

Harvard Medical Practice Study. *Patients, Doctors and Lawyers: Studies of Medical Injury, Malpractice Litigation, and Patient Compensation in New York.* Boston: Harvard Medical Practice Study, 1990, Technical Appendix 5.V.1.

Havas, M., et al. "Provocation study using heart rate variability shows radiation from 2.4 GHz cordless phone affects autonomic nervous system." *European Journal of Oncology* (2010) Library vol. 5: 273–300.

Helm, H.M., et al. "Does private religious activity prolong survival? A six-year follow-up study of 3,851 older adults." *Journals of Gerontology* (2000) 55 (7): M400–M405.

Heneghan, C., et al. "Ongoing problems with metal-on-metal hip implants." *British Medical Journal* (2012) 344: e1349.

Hicks, J.M. "Screening for cancer . . . a very big business." *Healthy Eating, Healthy World*, http://hpjmh.com/2011/02/21/screening-for-cancer-very-big-business/.

———. *Healthy Eating, Healthy World: Unleashing the Power of Plant-Based Nutrition*. Dallas, TX: Ben Bella Books, 2011.

Hippisley-Cox, J., and Coupland, C. "Unintended effects of statins in men and women in England and Wales: Population-based cohort study with the Q Research database." *British Medical Journal* (2010) 340: c2197.

Hoffman, J.M. *Hunza: Ten Secrets of the Healthiest and Oldest Living People*. Island Park, NY: Groton, 1968.

Holt-Lunstad, J., et al. "Social relationships and mortality risk: A meta-analytic review." *PLOS Medicine* (2010) 7 (7): e1000316.

Hölzel, B.K., et al. "Mindfulness practice leads to increases in regional brain gray matter density." *Psychiatry Research* (2011) 191 (1): 36–43.

Honig, L.S., et al. "Shorter telomeres are associated with mortality in those with APOE epsilon4 and dementia." *Annals of Neurology* (2006) 60 (2): 181–87.

Horner, J., et al. "Telomerase reactivation reverses tissue degeneration in aged telomerase-deficient mice." *Nature* (2011) 469 (7328): 102–6.

Houston, D.K., et al. "Low 25-hydroxyvitamin D predicts the onset of mobility limitation and disability in community-dwelling older adults: The Health ABC Study." *Journals of Gerontology, Series A, Biological Sciences and Medical Sciences* (2013) 68 (2): 181–87.

———. "Serum 25-hydroxyvitamin D and physical function in adults of advanced age: The CHS All Stars." *Journal of the American Geriatrics Society* (2011) 59 (10): 1793–1801.

Howard, J.M. "Longevity in Hunza Land." *Journal of the American Medical Association* (1961) 175 (8): 706.

Hözel, B.K., et al. "Mindfulness practice leads to increases in regional brain gray matter density." *Psychiatry Research: Neuroimaging* (2011) 191 (1): 36–43.

Huang, X., et al. "Consumption advisories from salmon based on risk of cancer and noncancerous health effects." *Environmental Research* (2006) 101 (2): 263–74.

Hyman, M. "Conventional medicine misunderstands the fundamental laws of biology," drhyman.com, http://drhyman.com/blog/2012/02/16/conventional-medicine-misunderstands-the-fundamental-laws-of-biology/.

Ivanov, V., et al. "The radiation risks of cerebrovascular diseases among liquidators." *Radiatsionnaiabiologiia, radioecologiia / Rossiiskaiaakademiianauk* (2005) 45 (3): 261–70.

Jacobs, B.S., et al. "Stroke in the young in the Northern Manhattan stroke study." *Stroke* (2002) 33 (12): 2789–93.

Jacobs, T.L., et al. "Intensive meditation training, immune cell telomerase activity, and psychological mediators." *Psychoneuroendocrinology* (2010) 36 (5): 664–81.

Jain, P., et al. "Commercial soft drinks: pH and in vitro dissolution of enamel." *General Dentistry* (2007) 55 (2): 150–54.

Jenkins, D.J.A. "Effect of dietary portfolio of cholesterol-lowering foods given at two levels of intensity of dietary advice on serum lipids in hyperlipidemia: A randomized controlled trial." *Journal of the American Medical Association* (2011) 306 (8): 831–39.

Jensen, T.K., et al. "Caffeine intake and semen quality in a population of 2,554 young Danish men." *American Journal of Epidemiology* (2010) 171 (8): 883–91.

Ju, Y., et al. "Sleep disruption and risk of preclinical Alzheimer's disease," presented at the American Academy of Neurology's 64th annual meeting in New Orleans, February 14, 2012.

Julander, A., et al. "Polybrominated Diphenyl Ethers—plasma levels and thyroid status of workers at an electronic recycling facility." *International Archives of Occupational and Environmental Health* (2005) 78 (7): 584–92.

Kalt, W., et al. "Anthocyanin content and profile within and among blueberry species." *Canadian Journal of Plant Science* (1999) 79 (4): 617–23.

Kaplan, R.M., and Porzsolt, F. "The natural history of breast cancer." *Archives of Internal Medicine* (2008) 168 (21): 2302–3.

Kennebeck, J.J. *Why Eyeglasses Are Harmful for Children and Young People.* New York: Vantage Press, 1969.This book is available at http://www.i-see.org/eyeglasses_harmful/. Website copy created and edited by Alex Eulenberg, June 2003; last revision November 30, 2003.

Klabunde, C.N., et al. "Cancer screening—United States, 2010." *Morbidity and Mortality Weekly Report* (2012) 61 (3): 41–45.

Kripke, D., et al. "Mortality associated with sleep duration and insomnia." *Archives of General Psychiatry* (2002) 59 (2): 131–36.

Krishnan, N., et al. "Loss of circadian clock accelerates aging in neurodegeneration-prone mutants." *Neurobiology of Disease* (2010) 45 (3): 1129–35.

Lam, V., et al. "Intestinal microbiota determine severity of myocardial infarction in rats." *FASEB Journal* (2012) 26 (4): 1727–35.

Lanctot, G. *The Medical Mafia: How to Get Out of It Alive and Take Back Our Health and Wealth*. Ryde, UK: Bridge of Love Publications, 1995.

LaRocca, T.J., et al. "Leukocyte telomere length is preserved with aging in endurance exercise-trained adults and related to maximal aerobic capacity." *Mechanisms of Ageing and Development* (2010) 131 (2): 165–67.

Leape, L.L. "Error in medicine." *Journal of the American Medical Association* (1994) 272 (23): 1851–57.

Levy, B.R., et al. "Longevity increased by positive self-perceptions of aging." *Journal of Personality and Social Psychology* (2002) 83 (2): 261–70.

Li, H., et al. "N-nitrosamines are associated with shorter telomere length." *Scandinavian Journal of Work, Environment and Health* (2011) 37 (4): 316–24.

Lichtenstein, P., et al. "Environmental and heritable factors in the causation of cancer: Analyses of cohorts of twins from Sweden, Denmark, and Finland." *New England Journal of Medicine* (2000) 343 (2): 78–85.

Lin, L., and Li, T.P. "Alteration of telomere length of the peripheral white blood cells in patients with obstructive sleep apnea syndrome." [In Chinese.] *Nan Fang Yi Ke Da XueXueBao* (2011) 31 (3): 457–60.

Link, A., et al. "Virtual colonoscopy; real misses." *American Journal of Gastroenterology* 98 (s9): S235.

Linke, A., et al. "Effects of extended-release niacin on lipid profile and adipocyte biology in patients with impaired glucose tolerance." *Atherosclerosis* (2009) 205 (1): 207–13.

Lowenthal, R.M., et al. "Residential exposure to electric power transmission lines and risk of lymphoproliferative and myeloproliferative disorders: A case-control study." *Internal Medicine Journal* (2007) 37 (9): 614–19.

Luders, E., et al. "Enhanced brain connectivity in long-term meditation practitioners." *NeuroImage* (2011) 57 (4): 1308–16.

———. "The underlying anatomical correlates of long-term meditation: Larger hippocampal and frontal volumes of gray matter." *NeuroImage* (2009) 45 (3): 672–78.

Lustig, R.H., et al. "The toxic truth about sugar." *Nature* (2012) 482 (7383): 27–29.

Macfarlane, G.T., and Cummings, J.H. "The colonic flora, fermentation, and large bowel digestive function." In *Large Intestine: Physiology, Pathophysiology and Disease,* ed. S.F. Phillips, J.H. Pemberton, and R.G. Shorter, 55–72. San Diego, CA: Raven Press, 1991.

Malkin, D. "Simian virus 40 and non-Hodgkin lymphoma." *Lancet* (2002) 359 (9309): 812–13.

Masi, S., et al. "Oxidative stress, chronic inflammation, and telomere length in patients with periodontitis." *Free Radical Biology and Medicine* (2011) 50 (6): 730–35.

Mazdai, A., et al. "Polybrominated diphenyl ethers in maternal and fetal blood samples." *Environmental Health Perspectives* (2003) 111 (9): 1249–52.

McCann, J.C., and Ames, B.N. "Adaptive dysfunction of selenoproteins from the perspective of the triage theory: Why modest selenium deficiency may increase risk of diseases of aging." *FASEB Journal* (2011) 25 (6): 1793–1814.

McCullough, M.E., et al. "Religious involvement and mortality: A meta-analytic review." *Health Psychology* (2000) 19 (3): 211–22.

McDonnell, W.M., and Loura, F. "Complications of Colonoscopy."

Annals of Internal Medicine (2007) 147 (3): 212–13.

McDougall, Christopher. "The men who live forever." *Men's Health,* June 28, 2006.

McGowan, K. "Can we cure aging? Controlling inflammation could be the key to a healthy old age." *Discover Magazine,* http://discovermagazine.com/2007/dec/can-we-cure-aging.

Meinig, G. *The Root Canal Cover-Up.* Ojai, CA: Bion Publishing, 1998.

Mertz, J.R., and Wallman, J. "Choroidal retinoic acid synthesis: A possible mediator between refractive error and compensatory eye growth." *Experimental Eye Research* (2000) 70 (4): 519–27.

Meydani, S.N., et al. "Serum zinc and pneumonia in nursing home elderly." *American Journal of Clinical Nutrition* (2007) 86 (4): 1167–17.

Mild, K.H., et al. "Pooled analysis of two Swedish case-control studies on the use of mobile and cordless telephones and the risk of brain tumors diagnosed during 1997–2003." *International Journal of Occupational Safety and Ergonomics* (2007) 13 (1): 63–71.

Morgan, L.L., and Philips, G. "Cellphones and brain tumors: 15 reasons for concern," http://electromagnetichealth.org/electromagnetic-health-blog/cellphones-cause-brain-tumors-says-new-report-by-international-emf-collaborative/.

Mueller, N.T., et al. "Soft drink and juice consumption and risk of pancreatic cancer: The Singapore Chinese Health Study." *Cancer Epidemiology, Biomarkers & Prevention* (2010) 19 (2): 447–55.

Murphy, L.R. "Stress management in work settings: A critical review of the health effects." *American Journal of Health Promotion* (1996) 11 (2): 112–35.

Murphy, S.L., et al. "Deaths: Preliminary data for 2010." *Division of Vital Statistics, National Vital Statistics Reports* (2012) 60 (4).

Navarro, E.A., et al. "The microwave syndrome: A preliminary study in Spain." *Electromagnetic Biology and Medicine* (2003) 22 (2–3): 161–69.

Newberg, A.B., et al. "Meditation effects on cognitive function and cerebral blood flow in subjects with memory loss: A preliminary study." *Journal of Alzheimer's Disease* (2010) 20 (2): 517–26.

Newman, T.B., and Hully, S. B. "Carcinogenicity of lipid-lowering drugs." *Journal of the American Medical Association* (1996) 275: 55–60.

Nison, P. *The Raw Life: Becoming Natural in an Unnatural World.* New York: Three Forty Three Publishing Company, 2000.

Northen, C. "Modern miracle men: Relating to proper food mineral balances." *Cosmopolitan*, June 1, 1936.

Null, G., et al. *Death by Medicine.* Edinburg, VA: Axios Press, 2011.

Oberfeld, G., et al. "The microwave syndrome: Further aspects of a Spanish study." Presented at an International Conference in Kos (Greece), May 2004.

Ohnishi, M., et al. "Dietary and genetic evidence for phosphate toxicity accelerating mammalian aging." *FASEB Journal* (2010) 24 (9): 3562–71.

Okereke, O.I., et al. "High phobic anxiety is related to lower leukocyte telomere length in women." *PLOS ONE* (2012) 7 (7): e40516.

Oman, D., and Reed, D. "Religion and mortality among the community-dwelling elderly." *American Journal of Public Health* (1998) 88 (10): 1469–75.

Osterholm, M.T., et al. "The Compelling Need for Game-Changing Influenza Vaccines: An Analysis of Influenza Vaccine Enterprise and Recommendations for the Future." Center for Infectious Disease Research and Policy, University of Minnesota, October 2012.

Ovelgönne, J.H., et al. "Decreased levels of heat shock proteins in gut epithelial cells after exposure to plant lectins." *Gut* (2000) 46 (5): 679–87.

Oz, M., and Roizen, M. *You: The Owner's Manual.* New York: William Morrow, 2008.

Pan, A., et al. "Red meat consumption and mortality results from 2 prospective cohort studies." *Archives of Internal Medicine* (2012) 172 (7): 555–63.

Park, M. "Diet cola drains calcium in women." CNN Health, http://thechart.blogs.cnn.com/2010/07/07/diet-cola-drains-calcium-in-women/.

Patel, S.R., et al. "A prospective study of sleep duration and mortality risk in women." *SLEEP* (2004) 27 (3): 440–44.

Paul, L. "Diet, nutrition and telomere length." *Journal of Nutritional Biochemistry* (2011) 22 (10): 895–901.

Pfeiffer, C. *Mental and Elemental Nutrients: A Physician's Guide to Nutrition and Health Care.* New Canaan, CT: Keats, 1976.

Phillips, E. *Kiss Your Dentist Good-Bye.* Austin, TX: Greenleaf Book Group Press, 2010.

Physicians Committee for Responsible Medicine. "Section three: When is surgery unnecessary?," http://www.pcrm.org/research/healthcare-professionals/medicine-curriculum/when-is-surgery-unnecessary.

Pietinen, P., et al. "Intake of fatty acids and risk of coronary heart disease in a cohort of Finnish men: The Alpha-Tocopherol, Beta-Carotene Cancer Prevention Study." *American Journal of Epidemiology* (1997) 145 (10): 876–87.

Poling, D. "Running man passes away: Jim Hammond dies in his sleep at age 95." *Valdosta Daily Times*, http://valdostadailytimes.com/local/x1155937321/Running-man-passes-away.

Pusztai, A., et al. "Antinutritive effects of wheat-germ agglutinin and other N-acetylglucosamine-specific lectins." *British Journal of Nutrition* (1993) 70 (1):313–21.

Puterman, E., et al. "The power of exercise: Buffering the effect of chronic stress on telomere length." *PLOS ONE* (2010) 5 (5): e10837.

Rahman, N.M., et al. "Investigating suspected malignant pleural effusion." *British Medical Journal* (2007) 334 (7586): 206–7.

Ramagopalan, S.V. "A ChIP-seq defined genome-wide map of vitamin D receptor binding: Associations with disease and evolution." *Genome Research* (2010) 20 (10): 1352–60.

Rapp, D. *Our Toxic World: A Wake-Up Call.* New Brunswick, NJ: Environmental Research Foundation, 2003.

Reed, K., et al. "Health Grades: Hospital quality and clinical excellence study." *Lancet* (1995) 346 (8966): 29–32.

Reffelmann, T., et al. "Low serum magnesium concentrations predict cardiovascular and all-cause mortality." *Atherosclerosis* (2011) 219 (1): 280–84.

Report of the Standing Committee on the Scientific Evaluation of Dietary Reference Intakes and its Panel on Folate, Other B Vitamins, and Choline and Subcommittee on Upper Reference Levels of Nutrients, Food and Nutrition Board, Institute of Medicine. *Dietary Reference Intakes for Thiamin, Riboflavin, Niacin, Vitamin B₆, Folate, Vitamin B₁₂, Pantothenic Acid, Biotin, and Choline.* Washington, DC: National Academy Press, 1998.

Richards, J.B., et al. "Higher serum vitamin D concentrations are associated with longer leukocyte telomere length in women." *American Journal of Clinical Nutrition* (2007) 86 (5): 1420–25.

Richardson, T., et al. "Molecular modeling and genetic engineering of milk proteins." In *Advanced Dairy Chemistry: Proteins*. P.F. Fox (ed.). London: Elsevier Applied Science, 1992, pp. 545–77.

Robbins, J. *Healthy at 100: The Scientifically Proven Secrets of the World's Healthiest and Longest Lived Peoples*. New York: Random House, 2006.

Rowe, W.J. "Correcting magnesium deficiencies may prolong life." *Clinical Interventions in Aging* (2012) 7: 51–54.

Sacks, F.M., et al. "The effect of pravastatin on coronary events after myocardial infarction in patients with average cholesterol levels." *New England Journal of Medicine* (1996) 335 (14): 1001–9.

Sadetzki, S., et al. "Cellular phone use and risk of benign and malignant parotid gland tumors: A nationwide case-control study." *American Journal of Epidemiology* (2008) 167 (4): 457–67.

Samitz, G., et al. "Domains of physical activity and all-cause mortality: Systemic review and dose-response meta-analysis of cohort studies." *International Journal of Epidemiology* (2011) 40 (5): 1382–90.

Sanders, J.L., et al. "The association of cataract with leukocyte telomere length in older adults: Defining a new marker of aging." *Journals of Gerontology: Series A, Biological Sciences and Medical Sciences* (2011) 66 (6): 639–45.

Sauve, S., et al. "Distribution and antidepressants and their metabolites in brook trout exposed to municipal wastewaters before and after ozone treatment: Evidence of biological effects." *Chemosphere* (2011) 83 (4): 564–71.

Savale, L., et al. "Shortened telomeres in circulating leukocytes of patients with chronic obstructive pulmonary disease." *American Journal of Respiratory and Critical Care Medicine* (2009) 179 (7): 566–71.

Savas, J. N., et al. "Extremely long-lived nuclear pore proteins in the rat brain." *Science* (2012) 335 (6071): 942.

Schairer, C., et al. "Menopausal estrogen and estrogen-progestin replacement therapy and breast cancer risk." *Journal of the American Medical Association* (2000) 283 (4): 485–91.

Schantz, S.L., et al. "Impairments of memory and learning in older adults exposed to chlorinated biphenyls via consumption of Great Lakes fish." *Environmental Health Perspectives* (2001) 109 (5): 605.

Scheibner, V. *Vaccination: 100 Years of Orthodox Research Shows that Vaccines Represent a Medical Assault on the Immune System.* Portland, OR: Co-Creative Designs, 1993.

Schnall, E., et al. "The relationship between religion and cardiovascular outcomes and all-cause mortality in the Women's Health Initiative Observational Study." *Psychology and Health* (201) 25 (2): 249–63.

Schulze, M.B., et al. "Sugar-sweetened beverages, weight gain, and incidence of type 2 diabetes in young and middle-aged women." *Journal of the American Medical Association* (2004) 292 (8): 927–34.

Sears, A. *The Fountain of Youth Breakthrough.* E-book retrieved from amazon.com, 2012.

Selye, H. *The Stress of Life.* New York: McGraw-Hill, 1978.

Seralini, G.E., et al. "New analysis of a rat feeding study with a genetically modified maize reveals signs of hepatorenal toxicity." *Archives of Environmental Contamination and Toxicology* (2007) 52 (4): 596–602.

Seralini, G.E., et al. "Long term toxicity of a Roundup herbicide and a Roundup-tolerant genetically modified maize." *Food and Chemical Toxicology* (2012) 50 (11): 4221-4231.

Shen, J., et al. "Genetic variation in telomere maintenance genes, telomere length and breast cancer risk." *PLOS ONE* (2012) 7 (9): e44308.

Shivapurkar, N., et al. "Presence of simian virus 40 DNA sequences in human lymphomas." *Lancet* (2002) 359 (9309): 851–52.

Simpopoulos, A.P. "The importance of the ratio of omega-6/omega-3 essential fatty acids." *Biomedicine and Pharmacotherapy* (2002) 56 (8): 365–79.

Singh, M., and Das, R.R. "Zinc for the common cold." *Cochrane Database of Systematic Reviews* (2011) Issue 2, Article No. CD001364.

Singh-Manoux, A., et al. "Timing of onset of cognitive decline: Results from Whitehall II Prospective Cohort Study." *British Medical Journal* (2012) 344: d7622.

Sjodin, A., et al. "Serum concentrations of polybrominated diphenyl ethers (PBDEs) and polybrominated biphenyl (PBB) in the United States population: 2003–2004." *Environmental Science & Technology* (2008) 42 (4): 1377–84.

Smith-Bindman, R. "Projected cancer risks from computed tomographic scans performed in the United States, 2007." *Archives of Internal Medicine* (2009) 169 (22): 2071–77.

Smoak, B.L., et al. "Changes in lipoprotein profiles during intense military training." *Journal of the American College of Nutrition* (1990) 9 (6): 567–72.

Stein, R. "Exercise could slow aging of body, study suggests." *Washington Post*, http://www.washingtonpost.com/wp-dyn/content/article/2008/01/28/AR2008012801873.html.

Steineck, G., et al. "The epidemiological evidence concerning intake of mutagenic activity from fried surface and the risk of cancer cannot justify preventative measures." *European Journal of Cancer Prevention* (1993) 2 (4): 293–300.

Strum, J.W., et al. "Stroke among women, ethnic groups, young adults and children." In *Handbook of Clinical Neurology*. M. Fisher (ed.).New York: Elsevier, 2009, 337–53.

Styner, M., et al. "Mechanical strain downregulates C/EBPbeta in MSC and decreases endoplasmic reticulum stress." *PLOSONE* (2012) 7 (12): e51613.

Sun, Q., et al. "Healthy lifestyle and leukocyte telomere length in U.S. women." *PLOS ONE* (2012) 7 (5): e38374.

Taira, K., et al. "Sleep health and lifestyle of elderly people in Ogimi, a village of longevity." *Psychiatry and Clinical Neurosciences* (2002) 56 (3): 243–44.

Testa, R., et al. "Leukocyte telomere length is associated with complications of type-2 diabetes mellitus." *Diabetic Medicine* (2011) 28 (11): 1388–94.

The Endocrine Society. "Fructose sugar makes maturing human fat cells fatter, less insulin-sensitive." News Room, Endocrine Society, http://www.endo-society.org/media/ENDO-10/research/Fructosesugar-makes-maturing-human.cfm.

Thomas, D. "Mineral depletion in foods over the period 1940 to 1991." *Nutrition Practitioner* (2001) 2 (1): 27–29.

Trumbo, P., et al. "Dietary reference intakes: Vitamin A, vitamin K, arsenic, boron, chromium, copper, iodine, iron, manganese, molybdenum, nickel, silicon, vanadium, and zinc." *Journal of the American Dietetic Association* (2001) 101 (3): 294–301.

Tucker, K.L., et al. "Colas, but not other carbonated beverages, are associated with low bone mineral density in older women: The Framingham Osteoporosis Study." *American Journal of Clinical Nutrition* (2006) 84 (4): 936–42.

Tudek, B., et al. "Foci of aberrant crypts in the colons of mice and rats exposed to carcinogens associated with food." *Cancer Research* (1989) 49 (5): 1236–40.

U.S. Office of Technology Assessment. *Assessing the Efficacy and Safety of Medical Technologies.* September 1978.

U.S. Food and Drug Administration. "Follow-up to the June 4, 2008 early communication about the ongoing safety review of tumor necrosis factor (TNF) blockers (marketed as Remicade, Enbrel, Humira, Cimzia, and Simponi)," http://www.fda.gov/Drugs/Drug Safety/PostmarketDrugSafetyInformationforPatientsandProviders/ DrugSafetyInformationforHeathcareProfessionals/ucm174449.htm.

Ulger, Z., et al. "Intra-erythrocyte magnesium levels and their clinical implication in geriatric outpatients." *Journal of Nutrition, Health and Aging* (2010) 14 (10): 810–14.

Valentine, T. "Hidden hazards of microwave cooking." *NEXUS Magazine* (1995) 2 (25).

Valero, M.C., et al. "Eccentric exercise facilitates mesenchymal stem cell appearance in skeletal muscle." *PLOS ONE* (2012) 7 (1): e29760.

Vallejo, F., et al. "Phenolic compound contents in edible parts of broccoli inflorescences after domestic cooking." *Journal of the Science of Food and Agriculture* (2003) 83 (14): 1511–16.

Velicer, C.M., et al. "Antibiotic use in relation to the risk of breast cancer." *Journal of the American Medical Association* (2004) 291 (7): 827–35.

Vendômois, J.S., et al. "A comparison of the effects of three GM corn varieties on mammalian health." *International Journal of Biological Sciences* (2009) 5 (7): 706–26.

Venkatram, S., et al. "Vitamin D deficiency is associated with mortality in the medical intensive care unit." *Critical Care* (2011) 15 (6): R292.

Verdelho, A., et al. "Physical activity prevents progression for cognitive impairment and vascular dementia: Results from the LADIS (Leukaraiosis and Disability) Study." *Stroke* (2012) 43 (12): 3331–35.

Vilchez, R.A., et al. "Association between simian virus 40 and non-Hodgkin lymphoma." *Lancet* (2002) 359 (9309): 817–23.

Vinson, J.A., and Bose, P. "Comparative bioavailability of synthetic and natural vitamin C in guinea pigs." *Nutrition Reports International* (1983) 27 (4): 875–80.

Visciano, P., et al. "Polycyclic aromatic hydrocarbons in fresh and cold-smoked Atlantic salmon filets." *Journal of Food Protection* (2006) 69 (5): 1134–38.

Vithoulkas, G. "Acceptance speech: Right Livelihood Award (Swedish Parliament)," http://www.vithoulkas.com/en/george-vithoulkas/alternative-nobel-prize/2175-swedish-parliament-speech.html.

Walford, R., and Walford, L. *The Anti-aging Plan: The Nutrient-Rich, Low-Calorie Way of Eating for a Longer Life—The Only Diet Scientifically Proven to Extend Your Health Years.* Boston: Da Capo Press, 2005.

Walker, M. *Secrets of Long Life.* Old Greenwich, CT: Devin-Adair, 1984.

Wannamethee, S.G., et al. "Height loss in older men: Associations with total mortality and incidence of cardiovascular disease." *Archives of Internal Medicine* (2006) 166: 2546–52.

Werner, C., et al. "Physical exercise prevents cellular senescence in circulating leukocytes and in the vessel wall." *Circulation* (2009) 120 (24): 2438–47.

Weverling-Rijnsburger, A.W., et al. "Total cholesterol and risk of mortality in the oldest old." *Lancet* (1997) 350 (9085): 1119–23.

Wikgrenemail, M., et. al. "Short telomeres in depression and the general population are associated with a hypocortisolemic state." *Biological Psychiatry* (2012) 71 (4): 294–300.

Willeit, P., et al. "Telomere length and risk of incident cancer and cancer mortality." *Journal of the American Medical Association* (2010) 304 (1): 69–75.

Williams, R. *Nutrition against Disease.* New York: Bantam, 1981.

Wilson, J.F., et al. "Balancing the risks and benefits of fish consumption." *Annals of Internal Medicine* (2004) 141 (2): 977–80.

Winer, E.P., et al. "Case records of the Massachusetts General Hospital. Case 32-2007. A 62-year-old woman with a second breast cancer." *New England Journal of Medicine* (2007) 357 (16): 1640–48.

Wolkowitz, O.M., et. al. "Leukocyte telomere length in major depression." *PLOS ONE* (2011) 5 (3): e17837.

Wong, L.S.M., et al. "Renal dysfunction is associated with shorter telomere length in heart failure." *Clinical Research in Cardiology* (2009) 98 (10): 629–34.

Wright, C.J., and Mueller C.B. "Screening mammography and public health policy: The need for perspective." *Lancet* (1995) 346 (8966): 29–32.

Wu, M.M., et al. "Dose-response relation between arsenic concentration in well water and mortality from cancers and cardiovascular diseases." *American Journal of Epidemiology* (1989) 130 (6): 1123–32.

Wyshak, G. "Teenaged girls, carbonated beverage consumption, and bone fractures." *Archives of Pediatric and Adolescent Medicine* (2000) 154 (6): 610–13.

Xu, D., et al. "Homocysteine accelerates endothelial cell senescence." *FEBS Letters* (2000) 470 (1): 20–24.

———. "Multivitamin use and telomere length in women." *American Journal of Clinical Nutrition* (2009) 89 (6): 1857–63.

Yamaguchi, M. "Role of nutritional zinc in the prevention of osteoporosis." *Molecular and Cellular Biochemistry* (2010) 338 (1–2): 241–54.

Yau, J.L., et al. "11beta-hydroxysteroid dehydrogenase type 1 deficiency prevents memory deficits with aging by switching from glucocorticoid receptor to mineralocorticoid receptor-mediated cognitive control." *Journal of Neuroscience* (2011) 31 (11): 4188–93.

Zehetner, J., et al. "PVHL is a regulator of glucose metabolism and insulin secretion in pancreatic beta cells." *Genes & Development* (2008) 22: 3135–46.

Zhang, X.M., et al. "Initiation and promotion of colonic aberrant crypt foci in rats by 5-hydroxymethyl-2-furaldehyde in thermolyzed sucrose." *Carcinogenesis* (1993) 14 (4): 773–75.

———. "Promotion of aberrant crypt foci and cancer of rat colon by thermolyzed protein." *Journal of the National Cancer Institute* (1992) 84 (13): 1026–30.

Zhou, T., et al. "Developmental exposure to brominated diphenyl ethers results in thyroid hormone disruption." *Toxicological Science* (2012) 66 (1): 105–16.

Zittermann, A., et al. "Vitamin D deficiency and mortality risk." *Clinical Nutrition* (2012) 95 (1): 91–100.

APPENDIX A

Foods with Acidic Effect on Body Chemistry

Food Category	Lowest Acid	Low Acid	More Acid	Most Acid
Spices/Herbs	Curry	Vanilla	Nutmeg	Pudding/ Jam/Jelly
Preservatives	*MSG*	Benzoate	Aspartame	*Table Salt (NaCl)*
Beverages	*Kona Coffee*	Alcohol Black Tea	*Coffee*	Beer Soda Yeast/Hops/Malt
Sweeteners	Honey Maple Syrup		*Saccharin*	Sugar Cocoa
Vinegar	Rice Vinegar	Balsamic Vinegar	Red Wine Vinegar	White/Acetic Vinegar
Therapeutic		*Antihistamines*	*Psychotropics*	*Antibiotics*
Processed Dairy	Cream/Butter Yogurt Goat Cheese Sheep Cheese	Cow Milk Aged Cheese Soy Cheese Goat Milk	• Casein/Milk Protein Cottage Cheese New Cheese Soy Milk	*Processed Cheese* Ice Cream
Eggs	Chicken Egg			
Meat and Game	Gelatin Organs • Venison	Lamb/Mutton • Boar • Elk	Pork Veal • Bear	Beef
Fish and Shellfish	Fish	Shellfish Mollusks	• Mussel • Squid	• Lobster
Fowl	Wild Duck	Goose Turkey	Chicken	Pheasant
Grains, Cereals, and Grasses	• Triticale Millet Kasha • Amaranth Brown Rice	Buckwheat Wheat • Spelt/Teff/Kamut Farina/Semolina White Rice	Maize Barley Goat Corn Rye Oat Bran	Barley Processed Flour

• Therapeutic, gourmet, or exotic items   Italicized items are NOT recommended foods

Foods wih Acidic Effect on Body Chemistry (continued)

Food Category	Lowest Acid	Low Acid	More Acid	Most Acid
Nuts, Seeds, Sprouts, and Oils	Pine Nut Pumpkin Seed Oil Sunflower Seed Oil Canola Oil	Almond Oil Seasame Oil Safflower Oil Tapioca • Seitan or Tofu	Pecan Pistachio Seed Chestnut Oil Lard Palm Kernel Oil	Hazelnut Walnut Brazil Nut • *Cottonseed Oil/* *Meal*
Beans and Vegetables	Fava Bean Kidney Bean Black-eyed Pea Spinach String/Wax Bean Zucchini Chutney Rhubarb	Split Pea Pinto Bean White Bean Navy/Red Bean Aduki Bean Lima or Mung Bean Chard	Green Pea Peanut Snow Peas Legumes (other) Chick Pea Garbanzo Carrot	Soybean Carob
Fruit	Coconut Guava • Pickled Fruit Dried Fruit Fig Persimmon Juice • Cherimoya Date	Plum Prune Tomato	Cranberry Pomegranate	

• Therapeutic, gourmet, or exotic items   Italicized items are NOT recommended Foods

Foods with Alkaline Effect
on Body Chemistry

Food Category	Most Alkaline	More Alkalin	Low Alkaline	Lowest Alkaline
Spices/Herbs	Baking Soda	Spices Cinnamon Licorice • Black Cohash Agave	• Herbs (most): Arnica Bergamot Echinacea Chrysanthemum Ephedra Feverfew Goldenseal Lemongrass Aloe Vera Nettle Angelica	White Willow Bark Slippery Elm Artemisia Annual
Preservatives	*Sea Salt*			*Sulfite*
Beverages	Mineral Water	• Kambucha	• Green or Mu Tea	Ginger Tea
Sweeteners		*Molasses*	Rice Syrup	Sucanat
Vinegar		Soy Sauce	Apple Cider Vinegar	• Umeboshi Vinegar
Therapeutic	• Umebosh Plum		Sake	Algae, Blue Green
Processed Dairy				Ghee (Clarified Butter) Human Breast Milk
Eggs			• Quail Egg	• Duck Egg
Meat and Game				
Fish/Shellfish				
Fowl				
Grains, Cereals, and Grasses				Oat Grain Coffee • Quinoa Wild Rice Japonica Rice

• Therapeutic, gourmet, or exotic items

Foods with Alkaline Effect on Body Chemistry (continued)

Food Category	Most Alkaline	More Alkaline	Low Alkaline	Lowest Alkaline
Beans and Vegetables	Lentil	Kohlrabi	Potato	Brussels Sprout
	Brocoflower	Parsnip/Taro	Bell Pepper	Beet
	• Seaweed	Garlic	Mushroom	Chive
	Noral/Kombu/	Asparagus	Fungi	Cilantro
	Wakame / Hijiki	Kale	Cauliflower	Celery
	Onion / Miso	Parsley	Cabbage	Scallion
	• Daikon / Taro Root	Endive	Rutabaga	Okra
	• Sea Vegetables (other)	Arugula	• Salsify/Ginseng	Cucumber
	Dandelion Green	Mustard Greens	Eggplant	Turnip Greens
	• Burdock	Jerusalem Artichoke	Pumpkin	Squash
	• Lotus Root	Ginger Root	Collard Greens	Artichoke
	Sweet Potato/Yam	Broccoli		Lettuce
				Jicama
Fruits	Lime	Grapefruit	Lemon	Orange
	Nectarine	Cantaloupe	Pear	Apricot
	Persimmon	Honeydew	Avocado	Banana
	Raspberry	Ciutrus	Apple	Blueberry
	Watermelon	Olive	Blackberry	Pineapple Juice
	Tangerine	• Dewberry	Cherry	• Raisin/Currant
	Pineapple	Loganberry	Peach	Grape
		Mango	Papaya	Strawberry

• Therapeutic, gourmet, or exotic items

APPENDIX B

Beyond Health® Age
Defense Formula

Inflammation drives the aging process. It is the foundation of every chronic disease. Unfortunately, because we eat an inflammatory diet, live in a toxic environment, and have stressful lifestyles, most of us are living with varying degrees of chronic systemic inflammation. This helps explain our unprecedented epidemic of accelerated aging and chronic disease. Inflammation generates free radicals, causing what is called oxidative damage. Oxidative damage to genes, cells, tissues, and organs is destructive to human health. When the oxidative damage exceeds your body's capacity to repair the damage, repair deficits are the result.

Repair deficits accelerate the aging process and cause the so-called diseases of aging. This is why virtually everyone needs to supplement with antioxidant nutrients such as vitamins C and E, carotenes, and selenium. However, even this may not be enough for most of us, because chronic inflammation tends to be self-sustaining, particularly in today's oxiding environment. This is why I created Beyond Health Age Defense Formula.

The Age Defense Formula is a powerful antioxidant formula that works at the genetic level to protect the body from oxidative damage and inflammation. Most chronic diseases and signs of aging result from free radical activity and cell damage. By signaling genes to upgrade their expression to suppress free radical activity, Age Defense Formula helps to slow and even reverse the aging process by minimizing oxidative damage and reducing the repair burden. Minimizing oxidative damage and reducing the repair burden allows the body to repair some of the old damage and protect against new damage.

The Age Defense Formula is a technological breakthrough. Highly protective against the effects of cancer-causing chemicals, it helps to prevent and suppress cancer, as well as all other inflammation-driven diseases, such as heart disease, diabetes, and arthritis.

To get well, stay well, and slow the aging process, we must first stop feeding the inflammation. Get off the inflammatory Big Four: sugar, wheat, processed supermarket oils, and dairy products. Avoid inflammatory toxins such as glutamates, food additives, pesticides, prescription drugs, fluoride, chlorine, and toxic metals such as aluminum, arsenic, cadmium, lead, and mercury. Address chronic infections in your gums, sinuses, and elsewhere; these create a constant flood of free radicals that do oxidative damage. Allergens must be avoided because allergic reactions produce a flood of free radicals—avoid the most allergenic foods like wheat, dairy, soy, and corn. Reduce your existing levels of stored toxins by taking saunas regularly. Control your stress with exercise and meditation. Just say no to vaccinations.

Once you stop feeding the inflammation, you have to work on shutting down the existing inflammation that has already taken hold in your body. Once established, chronic inflammation takes on a life of its own sustaining, but sufficient antioxidants can shut inflammation down. Anti-inflammatory supplements include: omega-3 fatty acids; vitamins A, C, D, and E; the vitamin B complex (including folic acid, B_6 and B_{12}); plus beta-carotene, CoQ_{10}, curcumin, quercitin, selenium, N-acetylcysteine, zinc, alpha-lipoic acid, and Beyond Health's Age Defense Formula.

Beyond Health's well-researched, revolutionary Age Defense Formula is primarily based on natural phytochemicals from food. It activates signaling pathways that initiate a variety of cellular events including the production of detoxification enzymes, antioxidant enzymes, and the expression of tumor-suppressor genes that inhibit cell proliferation and *angiogenesis* (growth of arteries to feed tumors).

To measure the antioxidant capacity of different foods and supplements, scientists measure the number of Oxygen Radical Absorbance Capacity (ORAC) units. Antioxidants combat free radicals, making an ORAC-rich diet a good defense against disease. Studies have shown that consuming fruits and vegetables with high ORAC values help slow the aging process in both body and brain. This is why the United States Department of Agriculture suggests consuming a daily intake of at least 5,000 ORAC units per day to dramatically lessen your risk of heart disease, cancer, and Parkinson's and Alzheimer's diseases. A serving of steamed broccoli contains 2,400 ORAC units, and a serving of fresh blueberries has 4,700. Beyond Health's Age Defense Formula has an astonishing 484,000 units in a daily serving—the highest of any supplement in the industry!

Because it combines high concentrations of powerful antioxidants with genetic activation of detoxification pathways, antioxidant enzymes, and tumor-suppressing processes, Beyond Health's Age Defense Formula can not only help to inhibit and reverse the aging process but also prevent cancer and other age-related diseases. Based on cutting-edge molecular biology, ADF is a product that all of us need and should be taking daily. ADF is available through Beyond Health International.

About Beyond Health International

Beyond Health International is an internationally respected supplier of supplements and health products of exceptional quality. Beyond Health's total commitment to quality puts it in a class of its own, offering outstanding value to its customers with more biologically active nutrients per dollar than lower-priced products. With supplements, high quality equals high purity and high biological activity, supplying your body with what it needs to get well and stay well.

Contact Beyond Health at:
www.beyondhealth.com
800-250-3063 (U.S. and Canada only)
954-492-1324

APPENDIX C

Green Schools
P.O. Box 323
Mansfield, MA 02048
Phone: (508) 272-9653
Fax: (425) 663-1757
E-Mail: info@projectgreenschools.org
Website: www.projectgreenschools.org

High-Quality Vitamins, Supplements, and Health Products
Beyond Health International
6555 Powerline Road, Suite 101
Fort Lauderdale, FL 33309
Phone: 1-800-250-3063
E-Mail: mail@beyondhealth.com
Website: www.beyondhealth.com

National Allergy Supply
1620-D Satellite Blvd.
Duluth, GA 30097
Phone: 1-800-522-1448
E-Mail: info@nationalallergy.com
Website: www.natlallergy.com

Restoring Oxygen Metabolism
Frank Shallenberger, MD
Nevada Center of Alternative and Anti-Aging Medicine
1231 Country Club Drive
Carson City, NV 89703
Phone: 775-884-3990
Fax: 775-884-2202
Website: www.anti-agingmedicine.com

Eye Exercises

Eyesight can be improved using natural vision improvement exercises. By regularly performing a series of simple exercises, most people can throw their eyeglasses away. Meir Schneider's *Yoga for Your Eyes* offers a complete program including a sixty-five-page study guide, eye exercise chart, and a seventy-three-minute instructional DVD that teaches you how to improve your vision naturally. Meir Schneider was born without sight. He developed his own total approach to self-healing and used it to reverse his own blindness. *Yoga for Your Eyes* is available through Beyond Health International at www.beyondhealth.com or 800-250-3063.

ABOUT THE AUTHOR

Raymond Francis, D.Sc., M.Sc., RNC, was at the height of an international career in management consulting when his health began declining. What began as fatigue, some chemical sensitivities, and allergies ended up as extreme chronic fatigue, extreme chemical sensitivities, allergic reactions to almost everything, fibromyalgia, lupus, Hashimoto's thyroiditis, Sjogren's syndrome, digestive problems, skin rashes, headaches, brain fog, dizziness, grand mal seizures, and acute liver failure. At age 48, his imminent death from liver failure was considered a medical certainty. "There is nothing more we can do for you," his doctors said.

Realizing that the medical interventions by his physicians had only made matters worse (It was a diagnostic test that plunged his health into sharp decline, and it was a prescription drug that precipitated his acute liver failure.) Raymond decided it was up to him to save his life. A chemist by training and a graduate of M.I.T., he began taking large doses of vitamin C, which revived him enough to conduct extensive research and direct his own care. It took him two years to restore his health to where he could function normally once again. During this period he developed his revolutionary Beyond Health Model of One Disease, Two Causes, and Six Pathways to health and disease. This is a model of health and disease that is so powerful that many thousands have used it to cure themselves of chronic and even terminal illnesses, yet it is so simple, it can be taught to a child.

Now at age 76, Raymond enjoys an extraordinary level of health. In the last twenty-six years since his recovery, he has not taken any medications or had any surgeries, and he has not been sick except for two colds. He is on a mission to reach as many people as possible with the message that you don't have to get sick and that "health is a choice." He has written four books, *Never Be Sick Again, Never Be Fat Again, Never Fear Cancer Again, and Never Feel Old Again. Raymond has addressed health conferences all over the U.S. and in six other countries and has made over 2,000 television and radio appearances. He is president of Beyond Health International, a supplier of health-supporting products and advanced health education.*

INDEX

A

Accelerated aging
  causes, 72, 74, 82, 99, 140, 150,
    155, 171, 172–173, 238, 278,
    321–324
as a disease, 8, 34, 62, 66, 138
and genetics, 275, 278
  improving symptoms, 25, 121,
    336, 339
  overview, 31, 166, 333
  prevention of, 68, 121, 232
in young people, 17–19
Acid. *See* pH
Advanced glycation end products,
    76–78
Aging
  Alzheimer's disease. *See*
    Alzheimer's disease
  beliefs about, 7–8
  biological age, 9–10, 25, 67, 123,
    149, 190, 232, 236
  choices and, 10–11
  chronological age, 9–10
  effects of, 8
  exercise and, 235–236
  health and longevity, 11–12
  life expectancy. *See* Life
    expectancy
  in long-lived societies, 13
  measurements of, 24–25, 27–28,
    47–59, 213
  and modern medicine, 286

premature aging. *See*
    Accelerated aging
  as a process, 8–9
  rate of, 8
Alkalinity. *See* pH
Allergies
  and acidity, 50, 57
  allergens, 95, 190, 374
  causes, 311
  and chemical sensitivity
    syndrome, 153–154
  resources, 154, 377
Aluminum, 164, 172–173, 315–316
Alzheimer's disease
  causes, 311
  overview, 15–16, 36
  prevention, 265
  treatment, 221
Angell, Marcia, 304
Animal protein
  alternatives, 127
  excess, 94, 99–101, 109, 163
  quality, 120, 149, 168–170
Anti-aging industry
  misinformation, 22–24
  products, 22–24, 321–324
Antioxidants
  Beyond Health Age Defense
    Formula, 122, 373–376
  overview, 122, 144, 165, 193,
    228, 308, 373–376